Acupuncture and the Life Energies

Acupuncture and the Life Energies

By Sidney Rose-Neil

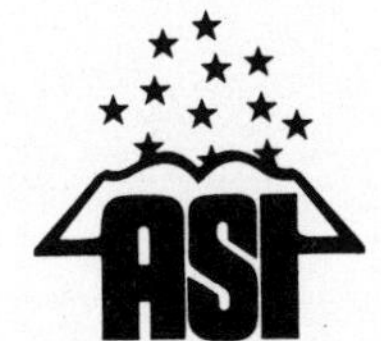

ASI Publishers Inc., 127 Madison Avenue
New York, N.Y. 10016

Originally published in England as
Acupuncture and the Life Energies

First American edition 1981 by ASI Publishers Inc.

ISBN: 0-88231-121-2

About the Author

Sidney Rose-Neil is the Director of Tyringham Naturopathic Clinic, and is also the Chairman and founder of the British Acupuncture Association. He is qualified as a Naturopath, Osteopath, Chiropractor and is also a Doctor of Acupuncture. Mr. Rose-Neil has travelled extensively to promote these traditional medical practices, lecturing all over the world, at universities, colleges and medical faculties. He has written many articles, books and papers on these subjects. He is a member of numerous associations working towards the promotion of Alternative Medicine.

Acknowledgement

My acknowledgements go to everyone over the last twenty years with whom I have discussed Acupuncture. Too numerous to mention by name, but to each and every one of them, I offer my gratitude.

A very special thank-you to my colleague, Royston Low, for reading the proofs so carefully, and giving so generously of his profound knowledge of acupuncture.

*Dedicated to my family
Pat, Sasha and Justine and the animals
who, by being quiet, made this book possible.*

Contents

Preface

I LISTENED WITH GREAT INTEREST to this series of lectures, and became fascinated by the way in which Dr. Rose-Neil gathered together the threads. His underlying theme, *energy, not chemistry,* in a sense obvious from the start, began to impinge itself upon my consciousness, as he expanded on it from so many varied angles, which I would never have thought of correlating.

He complained of lack of terminology for the subject, but this did not prevent him from getting over to us the immense wealth of potential sources of energy which we have available to tap as we expand our thinking.

Although I have practised Acupuncture for some years, many of the points he was putting over had not struck me so forcibly before: that mine was a profession which touched all levels of healing: the particular kind of responsibility which I was undertaking: and the value and precision of the philosophy under which I was working.

Seen from such varied viewpoints, I began to crystalize my own wider parameters, and began to realize that touch, magnetism, everyday diet, intuition, and so many more natural aspects could be developed at a knowing level, as part of my own personal system of healing. They could each be extended, and widen my range of the work.

As I felt my own depth of awareness expanding, I felt sure that others in the audience must have been having the same expereince, and I am very happy now to be a part of the further spreading of these ideas to those who could not attend these most rewarding lectures, by the extension of the lectures into print.

Norman Willis

Introduction

" . . . if the doctors would go on strike, there would be a health epidemic." — KASPAR BLOND, Brain surgeon and cancer specialist.

IN ALMOST EVERY COUNTRY in the world, Acupuncturists are now in practice, and, as a medical treatment, the use of the modality is developing at an impressive rate. Every day, more practitioners are graduating, and the numbers increasing. Standards vary from country to country, but the training received by members of the British Acupuncture Association in the United Kingdom, and now in Holland, is among the highest in the world.

The British Acupuncture Association, originally the British Acupuncture Society, was founded in 1962 by a group of practitioners who had obtained their first training in Germany, and wished to bring this knowledge to the notice of their colleagues in the English-speaking world.

In 1973, the Association became a registered charity, which enables it to accept tax-free covenant gifts, and to receive the benefits of bequests under wills.

In 1974, the name was changed from the Association and Directory of Acupuncture Limited to *The Acupuncture Association and Register Limited*, with memoranda and articles to give it the specific right to hold the Register of Acupuncturists. In 1977, the name has been further changed to *The British Acupuncture Association and Register Limited*, a significant step towards establishing and improving basic standards throughout the United Kingdom. The British Acupuncture Association is now the largest and most important association of Acupuncture in the Western world, its standards the highest obtainable outside the East.

The national policy of the Association is to seek official recognition for Acupuncture as a para-medical profession. Active steps are consistently being taken towards this goal.

The objects of the Association are to promote and encourage the study and knowledge of Acupuncture, which is a branch of medicine founded upon the principle that health is dependent upon a proper balance of vital energy forces within the body; to establish the status, regulate the conduct, and protect the interests of practitioners of Acupuncture (Acupuncturists), so as to promote and maintain in the public interest proper standards for the practice of Acupuncture; to establish, maintain and publish a register of qualified Acupuncturists, and to promote honourable practice; to exclude malpractice, and to decide all questions of professional conduct and etiquette amongst practising Acupuncurists; the promotion and encouragement of scientific investigation and research into the philosophy, technique or practice of Acupuncture, and to do all such things likely to lead to the integration of knowledge of Acupuncture, and to the growth, dissemination or improvement, thereby, of public and personal health and hygiene; to establish colleges and schools for education and training in the principles and practice of Acupuncture; to form, or otherwise acquire, and to maintain, extend and improve libraries, clinics, sanatoria, and the like, all services ancillary thereto, in pursuance of scientific research and education in Acupuncture, and the combat of ill-health thereby; to consider all questions affecting Acupuncture and Acupuncturists and, where desirable, to promote deputations; to petition parliament, and to take any other steps to press for, and secure, changes in the law affecting Acupuncture and Acupuncturists, in furtherance of the objects of the Association; to publicise the objects of the Association; to conduct appeals; to solicit, advertise for, or otherwise request, and to receive, hold, and make use of, donations or contributions *in specie*, or property of any kind, for the purpose of the Association, and in furtherance of its objects.

The Officers of the Association are all honorary, elected by the Members, and by the Executive Council.

Regular seminars are held to keep Members up to date with the latest developments in Acupuncture throughout the world.

The Association activities, courses and seminars are financed by the Members themselves, or by donations from the public, which are always urgently needed, to help to forward our goals.

The Association wishes to see Acupuncture available to all people who require treatment, without distinction or financial hardship. It is striving for paramedical registration by the Government, and legislation to ensure that adequate standards are established, and are maintained, and to see that the interest of the public is always paramount.

The British College of Acupuncture was set up by the Acupuncture Association in 1964, under its constitution, in which it is empowered " . . . to establish Colleges . . . and to award Degrees and Diplomas . . . "

In 1969, the close collaboration between the Acupuncture Association and Acupuncture Research Association enabled the college to move to London, in order to cater for the intake of students from all parts of the United Kingdom. Now, in 1978, the college, with its large teaching faculty, has students from many countries, and, currently, runs a branch in Holland, in collaboration with the Dutch N.W.P. (Naturopathic Group).

Thus, the Association, and its college, have strict ethical and academic control over Members of the Register, so that the public is fully protected.

From the foregoing, it can be seen that, in addition, the Association needs to stimulate research into all aspects of Acupuncture. It was for this reason that The Korth Lectures were introduced in 1973.

Leslie Korth, known affectionately as the *Father of Acupuncture* in this country, having been practising for over forty years, is now in his 90's. It was in honour of this revered Member that the Korth Lectures were established.

Walter H. Thompson was the Member elected to deliver the first lecture, in 1973. His title was *"As Far as We Know,"* a brilliant series of papers, the result of a great deal of research and preparation, excellently presented and documented, now available in printed form from the Association.

I consider it a great honour to have been asked to give the second Korth Lecture, and can only hope that you will consider that my own contribution is of value to you.

1　History of Acupuncture

. . . . Acupuncture, the traditional art, yet modern as tomorrow. Unless organized medicine immediately foregoes its usual grudging resistance to new ideas, it will forfeit, possibly forever, all hope of controlling the most promising field for critical research in this generation.

— WALLACE SHUFF, M.D.

THE ORIGINS OF ACUPUNCTURE are lost in history, but it is said that, as long as 7,000 years ago, it was noted, in China, that soldiers, wounded by arrows, sometimes recovered from illnesses which had afflicted them for many years. From such observations, the principle was evolved that, by penetrating the skin at certain points, many diseases were apparently cured. Later, it was observed that the size of the wound did not matter — only its location and depth. The Chinese then began to copy the effects of the arrow, by artificially puncturing the skin.

At first, pointed wooden sticks and thorns were used, but, later, bronze and iron needles were fashioned. By about 3,000 B.C., it had been observed that different metals produced different effects, and also that, in order to cure some diseases, it was necessary to produce a stimulating effect, and, for others, a sedating effect. The use of gold and silver needles was developed, as an answer to this need, since gold appeared to stimulate, and silver to sedate.

In recent years, it has been discovered that it is not necessary to use gold and silver needles to produce the desired effect, and stainless steel needles have become standard instruments — they are more hygienic, tougher, finer (therefore less painful), and they can also be produced in a great variety of lengths.

In China today, over 500,000 doctors practise Acupuncture; in Japan, over 30,000, and, throughout the East, the total number probably exceeds two million. In fact, throughout the world, there are more doctors practising Acupuncture than the number practising Western medicine. It is used in hospitals in many European countries, including Germany and France, and, in Russia, it is taught in several universities. There are now over 5,000 acupuncture practitioners in Europe. Its use is spreading throughout the West, and, in the United States, where hundreds of practitioners now use it, it is beginning to find acceptance.

The word "acupuncture" comes from the Latin words 'acus', meaning *needle* and 'pungere' meaning *to pierce,* giving a rough definition of "piercing by needles" or "needle puncture". It needs to be noted here that needle use is by no means all of Chinese Traditional Medicine, which is a treatment of the person as a whole, and includes moxibustion, again directly related to the points, and also diet, attitude, and way of life.

It is not known exactly when Acupuncture was first discovered, although it is said, in China, to date from the neolithic period. Apart from the *Nei Ching,* (which took 1,500 years to write) being finished about 3,000 years ago, other early records date from the Han dynasty, which lasted from about two hundred years before Christ to, perhaps, two hundred years A.D. The first bronze figure, showing meridian paths, was made in the Sung dynasty, about 1,000 years ago, and it was, also, in this period, that the first illustrated documents were produced. During the last dynasty, which extended from 1644 until 1911, Acupuncture fell into disuse in the main towns and densely populated areas, largely due to the introduction of Western medicine.

It was with the introduction of the republic, in 1912, that it began to regain its lost popularity, and, with the birth of the Chinese People's Republic in 1949, it really began to receive a new lease of life. A research institute opened in Peking, and medical students were taught these age-old methods. Western-type hospitals also began to use Acupuncture in their physiotherapy departments. Since this time, its importance has continued to grow, and, year by year, its use has become more widely established, culminating in the introduction and development of acupuncture anaesthesia in 1958.

A Dutch doctor of the East India Company, Wilhelm den Rhyme[1] was the first person, in 1712, to have brought any mention of Acupuncture to Europe. In the 19th century, Acupuncture was used in Europe for the first time, by a French doctor, Louis Berlioz. Acupuncture then became

---

1.   Rhyme, Wilhelm den *Amoenitatum Exoticarum,* 1712. British Museum, North Library.

very fashionable in France, and enjoyed a great vogue, but, because the practitioners were inadequately trained, it soon went into a decline, and was, before long, almost forgotten. However, it was another Frenchman, Soulie de Morand, who, in 1929, returned from China as French Consul, bringing news of Acupuncture with him, thus revitalising interest.

The facts upon which our knowledge of Acupuncture are based have, as yet, been empirical, and, up to now, most attempts to explain how it works in terms which will satisfy Western scientists, have failed. It is certain that there are forces working within the body — electro-magnetic vibrations, or radiations — controlling and linking different body functions. Research in various parts of the world is being carried out along just these lines, as will be discussed later.

According to the opinions of the old Chinese doctors, Ch'i — "the life-force" — could be described as *living electro-magnetic radiational pulsation:* it is the pulse which differentiates a live person from a dead one, the life force, the organic force.

If the circulation of Ch'i is broken down at any point, then illness develops. The sick organ may suffer from too little Ch'i, where it is blocked before entering the organ, or where it is retarded. This can be caused by trauma, when too much escapes through the skin surface; or by lax muscle tone, when the same effect will result. On the other hand, the sick organ may suffer from too *much* Ch'i, caused by tension or damming up within the meridians.

The fact that Acupuncture is thousands of years old can be said, by the cynic, to show that this form of treatment is based upon superstition, as it has not changed for 5,000 years, which means that there has been no advance in the traditional medical thinking. However, it could also be argued that, if it has worked and survived for 5,000 years, then it is reasonable to say that it will still work, and probably continue to do so for the next 5,000 years.

It is only when a form of treatment does *not* work, or the organism builds up resistance, or there are toxic side-effects, that it is necessary to subject it to change, which is often the position of Western medicine, where we have new drugs coming on the market every week. If the old drug works, and continues to do so successfully, why do we need a new one?

It must not be considered that health was ever the rule even in China, because as long as 3,000 years ago, we read in *"The Yellow Emperor"* [2]:—

"In former times, man lived among birds, beasts and reptiles; he worked, moved, and stirred, in order to avoid and to escape the cold and the darkness; and he sought a dwelling into which he could flee from the heat. Within him, there were no family ties, which bound him with love; on the outside, there were no officials, who could guide or correct his physical appearance. Into this peaceful and tranquil era, evil influences could not penetrate deeply. Therefore, poison medicines were not needed for the treatment of external diseases. Hence, it was sufficient to transmit the essence, and to invoke the gods; and this was the way to treat.

"But the present world is different. Grief, calamity and evil cause inner bitterness, while the whole body receives wounds from the outside; moreover, there is neglect against the laws of the four seasons, there is disobedience and rebellion. Evil influences strike from early morning until late at night; they injure the five viscera, the bones and the marrow within the body; and externally, they injure the mind, and reduce its intelligence; and they also injure the muscles and the flesh. Hence, the minor illnesses are bound to become grave, and the serious diseases are bound to result in death."

With a few altered words, this reading could be quotations from a modern textbook, or last week's *Lancet*.

Again, *The Yellow Emperor's Classic of Internal Medicine* [3] helps us to understand why this work is still regarded so highly in China, and also shows how Chinese medicine developed. In this passage, the Yellow Emperor asks his head physician:—

"I have heard that, in ancient times, the people lived to be over one hundred years, and yet they remained active and did not become decrepit in their activities. But nowadays, people reach only half that age, and yet become decrepit and failing. Is it because the world changed from generation to generation? Or is it that mankind is becoming negligent of the laws of nature?"

2.   Veith, Ilza. *The Yellow Emperor's Classic of Internal Medicine.* Page 149.

3.   Ibid. Page 97.

Ch'i Po answered:—

"In ancient times, those people who understood Tao, the way of self cultivation, patterned themselves upon the Yin and Yang, and they lived in harmony, with the arts of divination.

"There was temperance in eating and drinking. Their hours of rising and retiring were regular, and not disorderly and wild. By these means, the ancients kept their bodies united with their souls, so as to fulfil their allotted span completely, measuring into a hundred years before passing away. Nowadays, people are not like this; they use wine as a beverage, and they adopt recklessness as usual behaviour. They enter the chamber of love in an intoxicated condition, their passions exhaust their vital forces; their craving dissipates their true essence; they do not know how to find contentment within themselves; they are not skilled in the control of their own spirits.

"They devote all their time to the amusement of their minds, thus cutting themselves off from the joys of long life. For these reasons, they reach only one half of a hundred years, and then they degenerate."

With all the hundreds of years of advancement of Western medicine, could anything be more true of us to-day?

Further, Acupuncture, even 3,000 years ago, was not considered a comprehensive treatment, and its use, alone, was deplored. The Yellow Emperor was told[4]:—

"When medieval scholars treated disease, they used hot water and liquid treatment for ten days, in order to remove the five illnesses of numbness. (The *diseases of numbness* were those of the skin, the flesh, the muscles, the bones and the pulse.)

"When this ten-day treatment did not terminate the disease, they prescribed thyme and the roots of herbs. And when the stalks and roots did not show any alleviating effect, the topmost branches and the farthest roots, swallowed as medicine, were considered effective. The treatment today is different. It is not based upon the examination, as to the obedience or disobedience of the laws of nature."

4. *The Yellow Emperor's Classic of Internal Medicine.* Page 150

He went on to say that too much emphasis is placed upon Acupuncture, and that[5]:—

" . . . poor workmanship is neglectful and careless, and must therefore be combatted, because a disease which is not completely cured can easily breed new disease, and there can be a recurrence of the old disease.

"The most important requirement of the art of healing is that no mistakes or neglect occur. When the minds of the people are closed, and wisdom is locked out, they become tied to disease."

One of the earliest writings on the *vital force* again appears in the Yellow Emperor's *Classic*. Here the Emperor asks[6]:—

"When the body is worn out, and the blood is exhausted, is it still possible to achieve good results?"

Ch'i Po replied:—

"No, because there is no energy left."

The Emperor enquired:—

"What does it mean, there is no energy left?"

Ch'i Po replied:—

"That is the way of Acupuncture; if man's vitality and energy do not propel his own will, his disease cannot be cured. Nowadays, vitality and energy are considered the foundation of life; in order to keep them flourishing, they must be protected, and life-giving force must rule. When this force does not support life, its foundation will dissolve, and how can a disease be cured when there is no spiritual energy within the body? Good medical work is comparable to the topmost branch, or to a beacon. If these farthest roots are not reached, the evil influence cannot be subjugated."

Diagnosis in China was by the pulse. In *The Yellow Emperor*, we read[7]:—

"What constitutes a healthy person?"

---

5.   *The Yellow Emperor's Classic of Internal Medicine.* Page 150.
6.   Ibid. Page 152.
7.   Ibid. Page 168.

To this, Ch'i Po answered:—

"Man has one exhalation to one pulse beat, and this is repeated, and he has one inhalation to one pulse beat, and this is repeated. Exhalation and inhalation determine the beat of the pulse. Where there are five pulse beats to one respiratory movement, it means an extra movement is inserted, bringing about a deep breath of what is called a healthy and well-balanced person. A healthy and well-balanced person is not affected by disease.

"Those who are habitually without disease help to train and adjust those who are sick, for those who treat should be free from illness. Therefore, they train the patient to adjust his breathing, and, in order to train the patient, they act as an example.

"When the patient has one exhalation to three movements of the pulse, and when the cubit pulse indicates fever, one speaks of the *warm* sickness. If the cubit is not hot, and the pulse is slippery, one speaks of a sickness caused by *the winds*.

"When the pulse beats are small, fine and slow, one speaks of *numbness*.

"When a person has one exhalation for four movements of the pulse, it means that death will follow. When the pulse breaks off, and does not extend, it also means death. Uninterrupted, and regular, breathing is, to the healthy person, what a granary is to the stomach. This means that it is the stomach which causes a healthy person's regular breathing and steady constitution."

In old China, they had specific rules for the use of needles. It was taught, for example, that one should insert the needle in the lower part of the body, if the illness was in the upper part, and insert the needle in the left if the trouble was in the right. It was believed, at this time, that the acupuncture points were quite large, about the size of a pea. The needles were inserted through the patient's clothes. A sensitive point was discovered by pressure around the point, and the needle was inserted in the area of greatest sensitivity. The points were not considered to be exactly located, and the success of treatment was very variable. The practitioner would elicit a feeling of dull pain, and this form of diagnosis, by using pressure points, was, and still is, highly efficient.

Early in this century, Western medicine was officially introduced into China, and attempts were made to suppress traditional medicine. These were not successful, for traditional medicine is too deeply woven into oriental life.

In 1944, Mao Tse-tung gave his famous speech at a congress of educational and cultural workers in Tenan. He spoke of the need for the traditional and the Western doctor to combine their knowledge for the increased health and well-being of the people, in order to wipe out disease in the East:

> "Unite all medical workers young and old, of the traditional school and the Western school, and organize a solid front to strive for the development of the people's health work."

Since this time, traditional medicine has received a new lease of life, and the old and new now work side by side. Careful assessment is being made to establish which of the two medicines are best in which disease. It is interesting to note that, in a field where no-one would consider that traditional medicine would be at all useful, namely anaesthesia, it may well prove the anaesthetic of choice in the future.

2   The Philosophy of Acupuncture

A single needle may free the body from ten thousand maladies—

OLD CHINESE SAYING.

Confucius said[8]:—

> "To gather in the same places where our fathers before us have gathered, to perform the same ceremonies which they before us have performed; to play the same music which they before us have played; to pay respect to those whom they honoured, to love those who were dear to them."

The spirit which has come down through thousands of years in Chinese culture still plays an important part in Chinese thinking today. The Chinese have a great resistance to change and it is because of this that, when we study acupuncture, we must be careful to assess that which we can fit into our scientific approach to medicine and that which we must discard.

Many Western students of acupuncture fall into the trap of attempting to transplant Chinese ideas directly into their own philosophy. This is a mistake and acupuncture must be put through the same tests as any other medical subject.

Chinese culture and civilization go back thousands of years and influence is today slowly being felt in the western world, particularly since the recent exchanges began. There can be little doubt that this influence will be accelerated in the next decade.

Bertrand Russell once said[9]:—

> "I think that if we are to feel at home in the world, we have to admit Asia to equality in our thoughts, not only politically but culturally. What changes this will bring about I do not know but I am convinced that they will be profound and of the greatest importance."

8. Confucius *The Book of Rites*
9. Russell, Bertrand. *History of Western Philosophy.*

That was in 1946. He was hardly to know that, in the 1960's, Chinese medicine was to take a strong hold in Western medicine.

The Chinese are not usually considered an inventive people, but they had a form of shorthand over 2,000 years ago, were using compasses 1,200 years before Christ, making paper in the first century, and seismographs for recording earthquakes in the second century. They invented gun-powder in the 7th century, movable blocks for printing in the 8th century, and they had printed paper in the 10th century.

In the earliest times, healing was in the hands of magicians and priests, but, during the Chou Dynasty (1140 B.C.) these were separated, and the magicians became the doctors. This is not surprising, as the priest was mainly concerned with spiritual matters and clairvoyance, while the magician was concerned with more practical demonstrations and down to earth work.

Medicine today is still cloaked with magic and mysticism, and much of the awe which the average citizen has for his doctor is based upon this unfortunate history.

Religion and healing have been closely associated in most civilizations, and it was believed that fire, sun, moon, water, storms, stars and clouds were outward manifestations of gods. It was the task of the priest, magician and witch doctor to chase these demons away, and to placate them. China was no exception, and the three religions which dominated her were closely allied to these beliefs. Buddhism came from India about 67 A.D., and, within 600 years, it had become a very powerful sect. Faith-healing, hypnotism and auto-suggestion were powerful adjuncts to the religion. With Taoism, magic is the powerful cult used to frighten people.

The Chinese have a tradition of religious tolerance, and, in the old days, it was not out of order to follow all three religions, Buddhism, Taoism and Confucianism, at the same time.

Li Tan, who later became known as *Lao Tze* (The Venerable Philosopher), is said to have founded Taoism, and preceded Confucius by over a century. His life's work and beliefs have dominated Chinese thinking from the Chou Dynasty up to the present time.

Taoist thinking does not make sharp divisions between material and non-material, organic and inorganic, living and dead. One *eases* into the other, one comes from the other, and *is* the other in different combinations. Reshuffle one, and the other can be produced. What is different is the expression of the life force, the expression of its energy relationships.

According to Lao Tze, there are two cosmic forces, two basic principles through and around which everything evolves. These are the principles of Yin and Yang, the negative and the positive. Yin is the negative or *female* element, and, in its extreme, typifies coldness, disease, death and darkness. Yang is positive, and brings warmth, health, life and light. Their harmony gives us order in the universe, and disharmony produces breakdown. This underlying basic principle is in all Chinese art, metaphysics, crafts, religions, astronomy, philosophy, science, magic and medicine.

To understand how the doctrine of Yin and Yang developed, it is interesting to examine some of the great sayings of Lao Tze. The law of opposites both oppose and complement.

"It is when you do not dispute, that nobody in the world can dispute with you.

"All things in the universe grow out of something, which itself grows out of nothing.

"What is the softest in the universe can go against what is the hardest in the universe.

"The meek prevails over the strong.

"Blessed are the meek, for they shall inherit the earth.

"Nothing in the world is softer and milder than water, yet it can go against what is hardest, and physically the strongest, and never fail to vanquish it.

"He who covets fame, will exhaust himself; he who knows when to be content, will not be disgraced; he who knows when to stop, will not be in danger.

"The most innocent has the semblance of being guilty; the most clever has the semblance of being dull; the most eloquent has the semblance of speaking with difficulty.

"To those who are good, I would do good; to those who are not good, I would also do good.

"More laws there will be, more crimes there will be.

"Sincere words are not pleasing; pleasing words are not sincere.

"The good are not disputatious; the disputatious are not good.

"He who knows, does not know many things; he who knows many things does not know.

"The sage does not accumulate; the more he gives to others, the more he possesses."

As we are aware, the Chinese, in their philosophy, use the term *Yang*, meaning active and striving, and *Yin,* meaning passive and yielding. Yin is always predominant. This concept can be understood in the light of the above apothegms.

Lao Tze said "Yin the female element always conquers Yang the male, by being passive." Yin and Yang are the complementary, opposing, equal necessities in nature, and emerge as partners, neither of which can exist alone.

Yin and Yang form a monistic principle, and it is in this philosophy that Acupuncture has its roots — one principle, expressing itself as two poles, independent, yet complementary. One cannot be conceived of without the other; they fade one into the other, yet retreat from each other; they balance, yet each weighs the other down.

Today, it is understood that there is no real distinction between matter and energy, and the old idea of exact definitions in science is disappearing. Einstein, Whitehead and others have shown that the statics of Newton are, in fact, relative. Time and space cannot exist in isolation, but are expressions of each other, and can expand into infinity, or disappear into nothing.

There is no true static, everything is in a state of becoming. What is to become is in the future, and what has become is in the past. Everything relates, and nothing is permanent. Everything exists as a relationship, and nothing exists as a static, not even for a moment, because time itself is not static, and is but a relationship which is becoming.

There is no static, space or time, in pure science. All is in opposition, and all is complementary, in fact all is an expression of Yin and Yang. Life is a process of ceaseless becoming and decaying, non-living and living. Fundamentally, all is individual and timeless. The point at which Yang reaches its zenith is quoted by Lao Tze, as follows:—

" . . . therefore, the sage puts himself in the background, yet is always in the fore, remains outside, but is always here. It is just because he does not strive for any personal end, that all his personal ends are fulfilled.

"The greatest conqueror of man wins without joining issue, the best of men acts as though he were inferior."

From this, we can see the yielding way of Yang towards Yin, the giving up in order to get, the renunciation in order to gain. From here, with a little imagination, can be seen the follow-through into the more modern philosophy of eastern Zen Buddhism, the achievement of perfect Yang bodily balance with Yin.

In the old days in China, the sky, or infinite space, was considered the supreme Yin symbol and the earth the supreme Yang symbol. The sky, Yin, is centrifugal force, and the earth, Yang, the centripetal force.

Centripetal Yang produces the following phenomenon, heat — here we have the activity of the molecules — constriction, density, and heaviness, giving tendency to go downwards. By contrast, Yin, the centrifugal force, produces cold, which gives way to a slackening of movement, dilatation, expansion, lightness, and the tendency to go upwards, enlargement, tallness (in the vertical sense) and thin forms.

In the universe, everything has shape, colour, weight and movement. The lengthened form in the vertical is Yin, and the same form in the horizontal, is Yang. Yang is under the influence of the centrifugal force.

In considering shape, vertical forms are ruled by centrifugal force, while horizontal forms are ruled by the centripetal force. Although geometrically, they may have the same shape, they may still be antagonistic to one other—we can note that the horizontal yang centripetal form gives the appearance of being heavy and bearing down, while Yin, the centrifugal force, gives the appearance of being light and floating upwards.

Now let us consider colour. One of our first conceptions of the world is of light and dark, as, without this, we see nothing. The classification of colours into Yin and Yang is not difficult, the warmest colours being Yang, and the coldest Yin. Yang colours tend to give a feeling of tenseness, and Yin gives more the feeling of atony.

Colour therapy in medicine is based upon these observations, empirically, without understanding the significance of the homoeostatic, dualistic, principle of Yin and Yang. Colour in industry has been an entirely empirical development, for it was noted that workers felt better, kept healthier, felt more secure, and worked harder, when certain colours were used in their surroundings.

An understanding of the relationship of Yin and Yang will give an appreciation of all these relationships. The most neutral colours give a feeling of peace, because there is the greatest balance of the Yin and Yang principle. This is also true if there is a balance of Yin and Yang colours and shapes.

If we look into a prism or rainbow, or colours of the spectrum, we see the natural order, which fits this concept of Yin and Yang. At one end, Yin — violet. The colours run — red, orange, yellow, green, blue, indigo, violet. Colours near yellow, and approaching green, are nearing neutral, with green as the most neutral; on the Yin side, colours around blue, approaching green, are again nearing neutral.

Everything in the universe can be described in terms of Yin and Yang, by its colour, shape, warmth and weight. Even artists use this principle, imparting feelings of warmth, hate, love, beauty, escapism, colour, tension, relaxation, and other feelings, by their shapes and colours. It is easy to tell why a picture is warm, or cold, relaxing, appearing heavy or to float. Too much Yang colour will produce tension in the observer; too much Yang in the shape or form will give a feeling of heaviness.

In the West, artists do not really know why their pictures produce certain feelings, but, in the East, they do, as the artists understand, and use, the idea of Yin and Yang. This is the reason why, in the opinion of some people, the greatest art comes from the East.

We can look for Yin and Yang in all sorts of fields. Light, and other radiations, can be classified according to their wave-lengths. The longer the wave, the more the Yang, and here we have infra-red. The shorter wave-lengths go towards ultra-violet and Yin.

It is through the principle of Yin and Yang that the Chinese have been able to develop their medicine without the use of dissection. By careful observation of the function of living organisms in relationship to the Yin and Yang principle, the Chinese gauge the state of the health of the human organism.

The importance of Yin Yang balance is stressed in traditional Chinese Philosophy in human sexual behaviour. The Taoists believed the seminal fluid to be very precious, to be conserved as much as possible, and developed sexual techniques as a method of nourishing the life force, balancing Yang (male) and Yin (female), acting as indispensable nourishment to life-forms, essential for longevity, energy and vitality.

The Chinese claim that Yin and Yang, the two over-riding cosmic forces, give rise to the five elements – wood, fire, earth, metal and water. Everything – living, dead and inorganic – comes within the control of these five elements, and are all dominated by Yin and Yang. The body is composed of these forces. Such living things as trees are considered as bodies, and are therefore wood. Heat is included in fire, and therefore so are the warm-blooded animals.

The stuff of life is earth, from which the plants get their nourishment. When the correct proportions of the five elements are present in the organism, Yin and Yang flow in harmony and there is health. When there is disharmony, Yin and Yang are in revolt and there is disease.

The father of Chinese medicine was Shen Nung, who lived to be 140 years old, about 4,800 years ago. He is accredited with having written the *Chinese Herbal*, which enumerates 365 botanic drugs. There are legendary stories in existence about the old Chinese doctors and their great knowledge of the body, its functions and anatomy.

They used four methods of inquiry:– observation, hearing, inquiry and palpation. Palpation meant of the pulse alone and not of the chest. Hearing was not really auscultation, but rather a listening to the sounds of the voice. A strong voice was Yang, and a weak one was Yin. A hoarse voice indicated trouble with the heart, and a thready, fine voice meant trouble with the head. One of the most famous of all Chinese physicians was Pien Ch'iao, who lived in about 250 B.C. There are famous legends surrounding this doctor and his great knowledge of anatomy and surgery. He is said to have made two patients insensible with narcotic wine, probably containing hemp, and, while they were under narcosis, he opened their chests, removed their hearts and exchanged them. The patients recovered.

However, after the great progress under the Taoists, there was no further development for thousands, of years. The philosophy of both the Confucians and the Buddhists taught that the body was sacred, that it was wrong to mutilate it in any way, so prohibiting either surgery or dissection.

Even the Viceroy's Hospital Medical School, which was the first modern school of medicine, did not have a dissection department, and only occasional autopsies were permitted. It was not until 1913 that it became legal to perform dissection. But, although this may have retarded medical research, it did mean that it had been essential to develop other methods of diagnosis to a very high degree, based on the Life Forces.

From the *Yellow Emperor,* it is interesting to note that disease is divided into two groups — those which spring from internal causes, and include the emotions such as joy, grief, fear and anger; and those which spring from external causes, including food, dryness, moisture, wind and cold. Great importance is laid upon the influence of the season, and of atmospheric changes, but the most important method of diagnosis was by the pulse, and all other methods became subservient to this. The theory of pulse diagnosis is based upon the principle of the five elements, upon Yin and Yang, and an understanding of the energies within the body.

On the facing page is a diagram to indicate the relationship between chemical and energy influences, to show how homoeopathy, but also perhaps how the universe works, energy influence increasing proportionately to the lessening of material content, the basic tenet of the ensuing thesis.

Chemical and Energy Influences

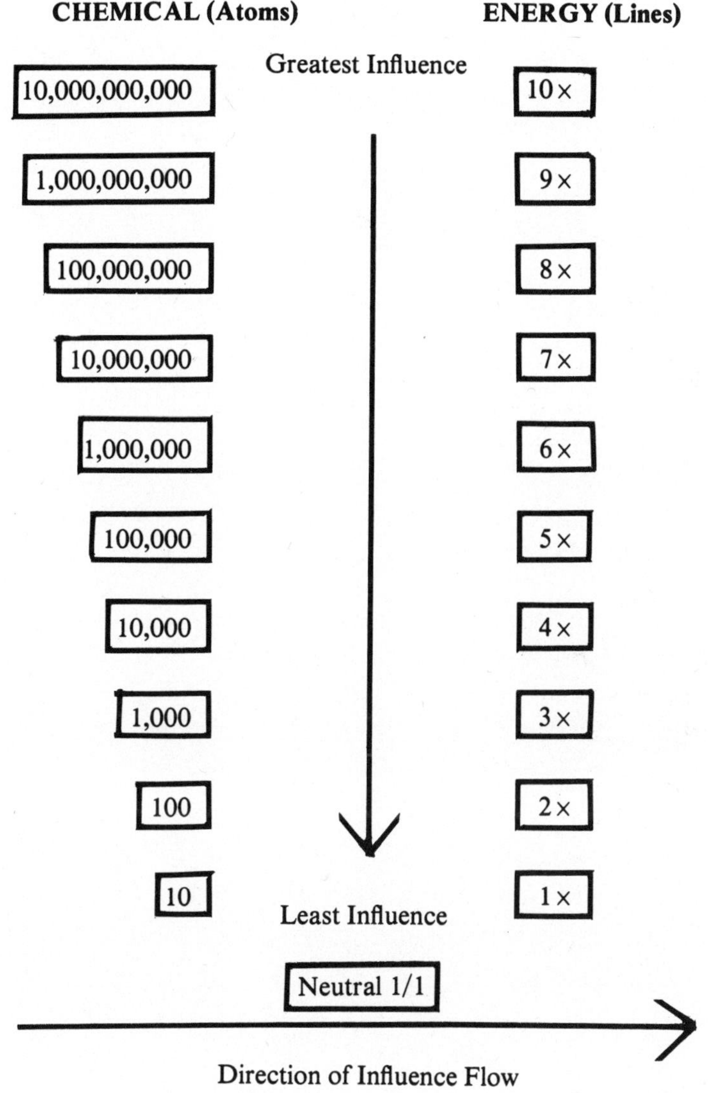

3 Orientation

One perceives the fundamental essence of life in the living, not in the inanimate, in that which is changing, not what is finished – GOETHE

FOR 250 YEARS, Acupuncture has been used by doctors in France, but it did not achieve a great hold on medical thought. After the war, this almost unknown but highly successful Eastern therapy was referred to, time and time again, in lectures at medical conferences, and in articles in medical journals. The consequence of this was the formation, in Germany, of an off-shoot to the naturopathic medical association, by way of a society and an academic journal. This society joined the International Association of Acupuncture, with its head office in Paris. With this increased stimulus coming from the German naturopathic doctors, Acupuncture received a new impetus in Europe.

Very soon, books on Acupuncture appeared in abundance in both German and French. While it cannot be said that the therapy is endorsed by the respective medical associations in the various European countries, the medical universities in Germany adopt a neutral attitude, and some universities in France show an unbiassed approach. It is only in the Eastern countries that there is official sanction for its use and development.

It is being discovered that the Pavlovian 19th century idea of a cortico-visceral reflex, based on an analytical-mechanistic system, is inadequate in explaining the complex relationships which exist in the universe. The effects and transference of energy and its relationship to matter, are forcing scientists to take heed of the functional theory of Wilhelm Reich. His work, together with the emergence of scientific verification of such age-old ideas as E.S.P., radionics, organistic-energy emissions, and others, are forcing us away from mechanism, and towards a basic functional approach; there being no other way to interpret, or to investigate, these phenomena.

Friedrich Kraus, of the Graz Clinic, in the 1960's, was the first to combine the regulative body devices such as the hormones, the vegetative nervous system and the physico-chemical system into the idea of a complete vegetative system. If we add to the work of Kraus the action of the electrical colloidal system in the organism, we may say that, in the vegetative system, Acupuncture could play an integral role.

When considering the work of Kraus, it is important to take into account the work of Vollmer, who, in 1923, at the Bergmann Clinic in Berlin, expounded and demonstrated a system of vegetative permutation. He made this discovery by injecting subcutaneously, 0.1 c.c. of physiological salt solution. After 15 minutes, there resulted a drop in the acidity in the urine. This acid drop lasted for three to four hours, after which it went back to its original value. This reaction occurred, even if the injection point was blocked with an injection of novacaine, which would mean, in terms of the cortico-visceral-mechanistic theory, that there should not have been a dissipation of the salt solution injection into the system. However, the acidity reaction in the urine still took place.

With the needle prick at the Chinese acupuncture point, a reaction takes place, an explanation for which becomes extremely difficult, if one is not prepared to accept Vollmer's suggestion of a *vegetative permutation*. This control reaction does not react only in a single direction, from a superior to a simple organistic system, but also from an inferior to a superior control organ. Therefore, a needle prick on a seemingly unimportant area of the skin may affect the liver, the kidneys, the lungs, the heart, or any other so-called *superior* organ. In this sense, there is no part of the body which is superior or inferior; all are equal, and there is an interdependence within the organism. In the words of Professor Bachmann[10]:—

> "There is no causal relationship in one direction, but there is functional circle, and this of great importance for the explanation of the effect of Acupuncture."

Acupuncture, therefore, works on the system as a whole; it is a holistic-organistic-functional philosophy, in contrast to orthodox medicine, which is concerned with diagnosis and treatment of individual organs, and systems within the organism. In this, we are at one with Hippocrates:—

10.   Bachmann, Gerhard, Professor, Dr. Medicine. *Die Akupunktur eine Ordnungstherapie*. Karl Haug Verlas, Ulm-Donau, Germany, 1959.

"All parts of the body economy form a circle. Each part is, at the same time, beginning and end."

This basic conception permutates throughout Chinese medical philosophy. The regulation of deviations of organic processes, in so far as they deviate from the norm, is the purpose of Acupuncture and this is brought about by a regulation of the necessary energy balance between Yin and Yang.

These disease deviations are brought about by one-sided non-compensated effects. The regulation of these abnormalities can initially swing past the norm towards the opposite pole. Here must be recognized the law of rhythm and polarity, which is a basic phenomenon of energy and nature.

With acupuncture treatment, we often experience over-reaction initially on either the sympathetic or the vegetative nervous system. With tonic or stimulating needling, as with sedative or soothing needling, we seek to regulate the energy balance between Yin and Yang. These therapeutic measures depend on the principle of polarity. Unfavourable results are often caused by a one-sided, too strong, energy effect of either Yin or Yang.

Chinese acupuncture theories are now having scientific explanations thrust upon them by research workers. Rusetzky[11] explains that we must take into consideration the embryonic stage of growth in evaluating heredity and environmental influences and in assessing health and disease, apart from the accepted traditional relationships of the segmental divisions and their relationships to the organs. Bachmann endorses Rusetzky's view, when he says[12]:–

"The transformation of the blastula and the gastrulation lead to development of the intestinal tube and the excretion apparatus of the organs attached to it. The whole of the hollow organs, with smooth muscles and strong sympathetic or parasympathetic innervation, belong to a particular system that is the Yang system. The Chinese have called them *Yang* or working organs and polar opposite are the *Yin* or the storage organs."

I wish, however, to offer a new viewpoint on Acupuncture and to show that the human animal is not just a collection of chemicals as science would have us believe, but an integral part with the whole of the cosmos.

11.   Rusetzky, J. J. Professor *The Chinese Method of Therapeutic Needling.*
12.   Bachmann, Gerhard, Professor *Basic Information on Acupuncture.*

It is my contention that Acupuncture works by manipulating both energy and chemistry. I would like to demonstrate that many spheres of influence are playing their part in modern healing methods, and to show that it is possible for Acupuncture to be unrelated to nerve impulse influence yet directly related to energy.

What, in fact, I want to demonstrate, is that all the new, *yet very old,* non-material forms of healing have something in common and are slowly beginning to overlap. I have little doubt that there are under-lying principles which will correlate every one of them into a logical whole in the not too distant future. As I see it, everything points to the influence and control of nature by *energy,* not chemistry.

Science is going through its most controversial period for over a hundred years. There is a mounting challenge showing that man and nature are part of the same integrated whole; that man may be an open-ended cosmic force, in constant, immediate and universal contact with the whole of the environment at all times. For example, Homoeopathy shows that the more minute the dose, the more the influence on an organism the dose has. (Refer Diagram, page 31). One part in a million, hardly discernible by chemical methods, is considered weak by homoeopathic standards. With the dilution at one part in a million million, the result is dynamic.

But for over a century, scientists have ignored the consistent results. Homoeopathy works because the dose is diluted *beyond* chemical influence and has entered the domain of energy influence. The finer the dose, the greater the potential, which is the precise converse of the chemical theory.

But, were science to accept this, then the whole of modern medicine would be seen to be based upon limited premises, with test-tube proof no longer considered conclusive.

Equally, science has ignored the teeming proofs of radiesthesia and radionics, even despite the fact that water diviners have been used by armies and radiesthesists used by the police to find missing persons.

How could it be possible for someone with a witchhazel twig to know where water is? How could someone with a pendulum find a missing person? In some way, waves are picked up and interpreted within the human brain. All information must be available.

Fish travel thousands of miles, even sometimes upstream, to return home'. Birds migrate across oceans and continents. Chemistry cannot explain these phenomena, nor even the conventional concepts relating to energy. But, to accept the principles of radionics would upset the whole structure of science as it stands.

The more we consider the qualities of energy, the more strange it seems. It can travel through a vacuum as light does and, by its very nature, it must occupy all space immediately. It has no mass and is not influenced by atoms, except possibly, under certain conditions, to be deflected by them. There is nothing to prevent its immediate movement across all space to occupy all space immediately. The mind boggles. How could it be possible to *restrict* energy?

Light is said to travel at 186,000 miles a second, but even this has been determined by molecule-mass intervention. My postulate is that the less the atom's friction, the greater the movement. Slow down energy enough and mass will be produced, transmuting energy to mass.

Science has ignored the work of Wilhelm Reich, (Chapter 12), although he did a great amount of experimentation to prove his theories.

Further, science has ignored Kervran[13], who has shown beyond any reasonable doubt that atoms can change from one to another without the use of any apparent chemical energy. The rationale behind his work would have revolutionized science had the authorities been willing to listen.

The brilliant lecture presented by John Wheaton[14] on ancient beliefs in relation to the earth's magnetic forces across the country and the building of monuments so many hundreds of years ago in perfect alignment should make scientists look up and listen and probe.

Extra-sensory perception has been dismissed. Psychic surgery, and the laying on of hands, have also been ignored as healing systems by the orthodox authorities.

We are led to believe that healers heal by *suggestion,* yet cancers are healed, cancers which have been previously diagnosed by X-ray and chemical tests.

13.   Kervran, Dr. Louis C. *Biological Transmutations.* 1972.
14.   Wheaton, John. Lecture to Acupuncture Congress, 1972.

Psychic operations are successful: often the patient has been cut open with a kitchen knife, having a tiny scar to prove it, and no longer has the fibroid which had been earlier diagnosed by X-ray and chemical tests.

Despite the evident recovery of the patient from a malady which had been diagnosed by orthodox methods, when cured, the disease is said *never to have existed*.

Kirlian photography, one of the most important discoveries of this century, the scientists attempt to dismiss as merely cold electron emissions, ignoring utterly the consistent stream of visual proof available.

Similarly, Yin Yang wholefood macrobiotic dieting is dismissed as cranky, despite massive evidence to show its effectiveness in improving health. The scientists tell us that white bread, meat and cakes are perfectly in order, so long as the right amount of 'calories for energy' are taken. Proofs abound to dismiss this antiquated concept.

As for Psychokinesis, it must be dismissed as inconceivable by a finite mind.

But Professor Taylor, Professor of Mathematics at London University, said at a recent seminar that these new concepts are so revolutionary that he really finds them impossible to accept; yet he has to accept them, for he has incontrovertible proof of them. He cannot accept, yet he must accept. Professor Taylor, says that they *must* fit into the known forms of science; he feels that he cannot accept that the new theories on energy have a validity, for, if he does, then the whole structure of science as he knows it, will topple.

Energy is the *absence* of matter, and how can one look at the absence of matter using means which are composed of matter. Scientists cannot accept that the new science must be demonstrated by *new* forms of experimentation and correlation, working on theories which are not demonstrable by the old methods, or by chemical means.

In the last few years, science has received two body blows from which it has not recovered—acupuncture anaesthesia, and the activities of Uri Geller. From these two scientifically unproveables, there is no escape.

Before the Chinese allowed their press service to release their bombshell information on acupuncture anaesthesia to the West, they had already performed 800,000 operations. Incredible! Impossible! But more and more western doctors, surgeons and people of influence have seen and confirmed these operations.

Acupuncture, scientists said, works according to Professor Wall's (Professor of Physiology at London University) Gate Theory. But this was manifestly impossible, both the nerve paths and even the direction being wrong. Professor Wall himself discounted the reasoning, and suggested in the *New Scientist*[15] that it might be hypnosis. But, as it works equally well on small children and animals, the hypnosis theory, as also the theory of auto-suggestion, became untenable. The Professor of Anaesthesa at the University of Rotterdam[16] suggested that it worked in the Far East because Chinese people do not feel pain in the same way as westerners. But by now, so many operations have been performed in the west that, I am sure, the Professor at Rotterdam could no longer hold this view.

For the first time in a century, the scientists have been shaken, some put into turmoil. To accept Acupuncture must mean a reappraisal of all known medicine and science.

Then came Uri Geller with his phenomenal activities. Dr. Ted Bastin, a world-renowned physicist, believes that Uri Geller is absolutely genuine, and Bastin has had a great deal of association with Geller. One by one, the greatest scientists fell under his spell. He astounded the authorities at Stamford University, and Professor Tiller, by his abilities. The American Government[17] put Geller through weeks of tests, under almost impossible conditions, but he came out successfully. Professor Taylor of London University was invited to the sensational first television programme in Britain in order to prove that Uri was a trickster. Taylor came away shattered and, in his own words as a scientist a 'much changed man'. For six weeks afterwards, he said, he hardly slept. Every known basic premise in science had been broken by Uri Geller.

The combination of the amazing feats of Uri Geller and the operations performed under acupuncture anaesthesia, have astounded and shaken orthodoxy. Science can never be quite the same again. As I see it, it has to change, ultimately, towards accepting that energy is all powerful.

15. Wall, Professor Pat. *New Scientist* 20th July, 1972.

16. Seminar on Acupuncture at the University of Rotterdam Medical School, 12th October, 1972.

17. Panati, Charles. *The Geller Papers*. Houghton Mifflin, Boston, U.S.A. 1976.

Uri Geller further astounded the authorities at Stamford University, and Professor Tiller, by his abilities. The American Government put Geller through weeks of tests, under almost impossible conditions, but he came out successfully.

The combination of the amazing feats of Uri Geller and the operations performed under acupuncture anaesthesia, have astounded and shaken orthodoxy. Science can never be quite the same again. As I see it, it has to change, ultimately, towards accepting that energy is all powerful.

17.   Panati, Charles. *The Geller Papers.* Houghton Mifflin, Boston, U.S.A. 1976.

4 Energy

There are no miracles, only unknown laws. – SAINT AUGUSTINE

BASED UPON MY BELIEF that Acupuncture is more associated with energy than chemistry, let us consider the atom. It is the smallest single unit of chemistry known to be complete in itself. According to science, it is stable, and its structure cannot be disturbed so as to become another element, unless it is blasted by atomic fusion or fission. This takes tremendous power.

Dr. Kervran[18] has proved that atoms *can alter their structure,* and become other elements, with almost no release of energy.

Let us use the premise that energy is a basic wave form, which is *pre-matter* and therefore *pre-atom.* Atoms are basic to chemistry, but not necessarily to function. We are more than the sum total of our atoms. For example, with a biopsy, the moment a cutting is removed from the organism, its function is altered, although its atoms remain the same. The atoms in the animal or plant organism are balanced in such a way that it works almost in spite of its atomic make-up, and not because of it. The moment we take something away from the whole, it is no longer the same, and cannot function as before. Put the atoms in a different order, and the overall structural integrity has been destroyed, and cannot be recovered. The whole is more than the sum of its parts.

Every part of the body is integrated, working together in such a way that, in emergency, the lesser subordinates its needs to the greater. The structure is built up in such a way that each ascending part looks upward towards the good of the larger unit. Survival of the organism is the deciding factor.

Premising that the atom is a separate structure, with its own unity and completeness, how can it communicate danger or thought or feeling to its next-door atom? It obviously can not. It is equally obvious that, in Nature, there is nothing random. Some form of communication *must* exist, some link between atoms.

18.   Kervan, Dr. Louis. *Biological Transmutations.*

So, let us break free from the confines of only an atomic relationship within the organism. Why cannot Acupuncture be concerned with that which is far more basic than the atom, the energy-forms which must exist, which must in some way control atomic structure, movement and characteristics?

Modern scientific ideas concerning the atom explain very little in this respect. For example, they do not explain why a piece of wood cut in two remains in two pieces: why they do not knit together again when placed together.

Was it possible to separate each individual atom, formerly related in that piece of wood? No, it is known that the atoms were not touching in the first place. Each atom is separate, moving towards and away from each other at a tremendous rate, never touching or stuck together, yet holding together with power and strength.

Why do they no longer relate after a saw and a cut? According to science, it cannot be the atoms which caused the break, because the atoms are nothing over and above themselves and, in any case, they do not touch. They are exactly the same in the one piece of wood and in two pieces of wood.

So we can only conclude that there must be some other power which holds them together and keeps them apart. There is no point in pursuing the answer in the world of the atom for, as we begin to investigate, it becomes more satis-factory to consider *energy* as the explanation.

Atoms are so small that three thousand million could be fitted into the eye of a needle, as many atoms as there are people in the world. Each atom consists of many parts, considered to be the solid part of the atom. But even the 'solid' part is not solid and is composed of many parts.

The apparently solid part of the atom may only be a hundred thousand millionth part of the total space occupied by the atom. There is no reason to suppose that any object is solid, as its solid components are such a minute proportion of the whole.

What, in fact, gives the appearance of solidity is the speed of the movement of the atom itself. An electron spin-off from an atom could well travel several times around the world in a second. The atom itself is moving at this tremendous rate. How many times a second must each atom be moving towards and away from its neightbouring atom? Trillions and trillions of times.

Even within the atom itself, the individual parts are moving at possibly hundreds of thousands of miles a second, the electron maintaining a constant distance from the nucleus. Man may work to a millionth of a centimetre and we are rightly proud of our achievements. But with Nature working to hundreds of thousands of millions of billions of trillionths of a centimetre, within each atom and within each molecule, with unswerving accuracy and no fuss, there has to be an over-riding motivating power.

It would seem that the control of everything is related to energy, not chemistry. Any object attempting to penetrate this tremendous oscillation would meet, to all intents and purposes, a solid wall. The speed of movement means that each atom occupies every part of its own orbit trillions of times a second, so fast that it appears solid. It is here and there at one and the same time. Only something moving at an even greater speed would have a chance of penetration, which is in fact what happens in Nature all the time, with trillions of particles hitting the earth from the cosmos every second, moving so fast that they pass through all the atoms of the earth without hitting anything at all. Non-solid particles, in this way give the appearance of solidity.

Necessarily, therefore, bodies are mainly space and only one millionth part solid. Empty space, no. Something has to keep the atoms apart, to keep them moving, to stop them hitting into each other, to keep them in a confined space, to regulate the orbit of their oscillation, to keep the atomic parts at a constant distance from each other, to keep them rotating precisely, to keep the centre nucleus as the centre nucleus. This is energy, vibration, a wave-form electro-magnetic force, radiation. These forces must be extremely powerful and yet simple, gentle, a form of caring and loving, by their very nature more powerful than the atoms with which they are associated, for they control the atoms. The atoms cannot exercise control over themselves because the atom is controlled by its own nature and there is no way that it can control something outside itself.

There really is no language to discuss further the many forms of energy which may exist, perhaps a thousand different forms of energy. This is one of the main difficulties when discussing energy, that there are no valid terms available. We use terms such as magnetism, electro-magnetic forces, static electricity, radiation, waves, orgone-energy, prana, Ch'i, vital-force, etc. But what is needed is an entirely new series of words specifically to describe the various manifestations of energy.

How is it possible to investigate energy by using normal scientific methods, for at the very moment that we examine it in any way, that act alters its function, which is the manifestation of energy. How can the *absence* of matter, i.e. energy, have a structure or anatomy, for energy is the absence of these very things? In order to investigate energy, it will become necessary to evolve a new form of science, a form of *functional* science as Reich calls it. All forms of present-day science investigate by interference with function, by definition self-defeating in relation to energy.

The necessary interference is difficult enough when investigating ordinary chemical phenomena, but at least chemicals have form, weight and mass. But energy is weightless, massless, formless, as far as we know. Were it to take on a shape and mass, it would no longer be true energy.

There may be states of non-atoms which are not true energy, a form of *pre-atom post-energy*. But how is it possible to investigate true energy when it can only be distinguished by its function and not by its anatomy, and if any investigation alters function? At the moment, it is an insoluble Chinese puzzle.

When considering the investigation of energy, there is still a further problem. Given that we cannot use matter to investigate energy, as energy has as a characteristic the *absence* of matter, how can we look at something which cannot be seen *with* something. This is a dichotomy which science has yet to solve. We may only ever be able to look at the *functions* of energy, never at energy itself. Further, energy is only discerned by function, and even the act of observation alters it.

The most complicated piece of apparatus in nature is the body of a man, yet it is the most simple to investigate, for the observation and investigation appear to damage man very little. But when we enter the world below the atom, energy, Nature's most simple form, we find that it becomes impossible to investigate anything, only to observe and to postulate, for even the act of laboratory observation may interfere and change the pattern of that which is being investigated. Is it in any other way possible to investigate energy?

Let us consider another aspect. Are we contained in our bodies? If only one millionth part of our bodies is solid and the rest space-energy, we must be more in contact with the outside environment than with our own bodies, or is energy stabilized in controlled patterns as the atom is? There must, of course, be laws relating to energy.

I would postulate that the speed of energy is controlled by the friction produced by atomic movements which lie in its path. The speed of energy is infinite, and retarded directly proportionally to the density of the atoms in its path.

If the speed of energy is infinite, then it follows that energy, if allowed to travel without encumbrance, will reach all space immediately, and all energy will occupy all space immediately. There must therefore be no limitation to the number of energy waves which occupy space.

It is possible to consider that energy may, under pressure, produce a density which forms itself into transmutical atomic-like structure. As density increases, it could form into atoms. It is a possibility that atoms may be a form of energy-condensation and the relationship between energy and matter one of degree rather than an absolute. A continuous process of energy to matter and matter to energy.

If we consider our brain, can it be confined within a skull? Does it have to be so confined? Only one millionth part of the brain is solid, the rest energy, in open communication with the cosmos, receiving wave-forms, and giving them off, trillions of times per second. Why cannot the brain pick up vibrations from other people, and transform them into tough patterns? This is extra-sensory perception. All people are giving off vibrations from the brain, a two-way communication receiving and transmitting. We have lost the ability to recognize these vibrations. Speech has superseded the need to use E.S.P., but it is still there deep inside. It is used as part of their daily lives by birds and fishes.

As people therefore, we can assume that we are more in communication with the cosmos than with our own bodies, only a small part being matter.

Energy is in constant, immediate and complete communication with the total environment. That which stops us from feeling or knowing this, is our inability to pick up the vibrations. Some people pick up more vibrations than others. We can all learn to improve our ability, however, to enhance our E.S.P. Most of us have many unusual experiences, but tend to ignore them. By doing so, we lessen our ability to discern the experiences.

One interesting energy phenomenon is the story relating to the Cheops pyramid at Giza, which housed the Pharaoh Khufa's body in about 3,000 B.C. called the *Great Pyramid*. Bovis[19], a Frenchman, found some garbage cans some time ago in the Pharaoh's chamber, and other material which would normally have rotted, including a cat and other small animals which had died there. It was very humid in the chamber but, to Bovis' surprise, the animals had not decayed in the usual way but had dried, like a mummy. Bovis built a replica of the pyramid, and put into it a dead cat. It, also, became mummified. After much research, Bovis concluded that it was the pyramid shape, and gravitational location, that produced dehydration rather than decay.

A Prague radio engineer named Karel Durbal[20] subsequently did a series of experiments and concluded that there is a close connection between the shape of the pyramid, the directional position and the whole biological process of life. He came to the conclusion that, under the exact Cheops conditions, many forms of matter can be retarded from decay. He, further, found that a used razor blade, placed in the pyramid, became sharp again. He patented this idea in Prague in 1959, after opposition from the Prague Patent Office until he had proved that it actually worked. He called it the *Cheops Pyramid Razor Blade Sharpener*.

Razor-blade steel is a form of crystal, and crystal-like living tissue can reproduce itself. The edge of the razor blade is only one crystal-layer thick. As the blade is used, this layer rubs off, and the blade becomes blunt. As crystals can reproduce themselves, there is no reason why, in the necessary space of time, they cannot reproduce. This process appears to be enhanced by the pyramid, and, within a week, the blade is fit to use again. When making a pyramid, the precise proportions are essential — four isosceles triangles, hardboard or plywood. The base must be 15.7 units, and the sides 14.94 units. The stand is 3.33 units high, to stand the object on. When using the pyramid, the base line should face exactly north-south and east-west. If it is intended to test on a razor-blade the retarding of decay, then the razor-blade should face east and west.

19.   Ostrander and Schroeder, *Psychic Discoveries Behind the Iron Curtain.* Page 366.
20.   Ostrander and Schroeder. Ibid. Page 368.

An intriguing phenomenon perplexed a scientific team from the United States and from the Ein Shams University of Egypt in 1968. The team X-rayed Chephren, a sister pyramid to Cheops, in the search for new vaults, by measuring the amount of cosmic ray penetration. In theory, the more hollow the area, the more the number of rays which would penetrate, and the greater the reading in the seismograph. But, after six months, the scientists had to admit defeat.

During twenty-four hours every day, the I.B.M. 1130 computers had been working and recording. The results, when analysed, made no sense at all. Readings taken from the same machine at the same place, on successive days, produced entirely different readings. The scientists said that this was impossible, that it could not happen, but it did. The powerful energy waves in the pyramid obviously over-rode any other readings.

This story underlines the contention that there are other factors apart from structure, when considering energy, which may explain how Acupuncture works. Further concepts of energy are emerging so fast, and in such variety, from a number of diverse authorities conducting extensive research.

Everything is pointing science *away* from structure, and towards energy – what we know as *Ch'i*. The concepts of Yin and Yang and Ch'i energy are beginning to make sense in modern science, explaining what happens when a practitioner tells a patient to *relax and let the needles help tune into the inner energy, and even feel the flow of energy.*

5 Orientation Two

It has been said that, in order to discover things, one must be ignorant—
CLAUDE BERNARD, French Neurologist

IT IS NOT DIFFICULT to see how Acupuncture could become very influential in the last quarter of the twentieth century. In talking to the average General Practitioner, one inevitably finds that he is disturbed with the results of his work. He cannot give the attention he wishes to the patient. In a way, he has built his own prison, looking almost with longing at the Acupuncturist who is medically free and obviously achieving what appear to be miracles.

"If only I had the time" is the cry of doctor after doctor with whom I have spoken. "Even if I did the training, how could I put it into practice within the health service, with so little time with each patient". For years, the non-orthodox practitioner has been struggling: the naturopath, the osteopath, the chiropractor, the radiesthesist and others. But they have built up no statistics of their results. They have had no China, with eight hundred million people who say "it works, and we have performed thousands of operations using acupuncture, instead of costly anaesthetics."

Acupuncture fits in with the vitalist theory, with the homoeopath, radionic and healing practice, and now we find the new psychotherapists, the *avant-garde* psychologists, the encounter group workers, the Gestalt therapists, practitioners of psychosynthesis, of Rolfing, of awareness massage, of Reich, of co-counselling, all in tune with us.

Already, the Reichen masseurs and the awareness masseurs are using a form of finger-tip acupuncture massage. The eyes of the non-orthodox world are upon us. They recognize that our work fits into their work, and that we have the limelight at the moment. We are the trail blazers, we hold the key. It is a great responsibility, which must not be taken lightly. We must support the non-orthodox world which has been working for years in the field of energy and has been consistently saying that the body is not simply a combination of atoms.

Health is the balance between the physical, the emotional and spiritual. In some strange way, Acupuncture helps to restore that balance. And nearly all the non-orthodox medical methods are involved in attempting to do the same thing – Lakhovsky, Eeman, psychic healers, absent healers, Kervran, Reich, and the host of other pioneers. They have all been working along similar lines, by stimulating different parts of the organism in a way which seeks to balance the physical, mental and spiritual being. This may be expressed in many ways, but they must be free and at peace, in harmony, for the three spheres to be in balance. Health is the result of flow, harmony, balance, peace, a form of love and care, within the three inseparables – the physical, the mental and the spiritual.

This is the exact goal of relaxation classes, meditation, yoga, a Gestalt group, co-counselling, Reich and Rolfing. It is what the psychic healers attempt to do, and spiritual healers. Each approaches the same problem from a different angle. Some attempt to solve it mainly from the physical side, such as the naturopath or the macro-biotic student. They believe that correct nutrition will balance the internal forces, which will, in turn, balance the mental and the spiritual forces. The new forms of psychotherapy – co-counselling, psychosynthesis, Gestalt, and encounter – approach the problem from the emotional viewpoint, believing that, if the emotions are in balance, then many other problems, physical and spiritual, will be resolved. The absent healer works purely through the spiritual, believing that, from the spiritual, all else emanates. Bring harmony to the spiritual being, and the physical and the emotional will become balanced.

Krishnamurti works through the emotional, to produce a state of complete awareness within the being, so that the spiritual is freed, together with the mental, reaching a perfect state of freedom, complete inner freedom, of peace, love, caring, of complete letting go, without attachment. *To love is to be free* says Krishnamurti[22]. You cannot hold on to that which you love, for, to hold on to it means that it cannot be free. Where there is attachment, there is no freedom. We must become completely free within ourselves, and thereby we give all others freedom around us, which brings the physical and the emotional into harmony, and thus into health.

22.   Krishnamurti, J. *The First and Last Freedom* (and other works).
         Victor Gollancz, London, 1972.

It follows that, if the body is to be free and flourish, all that enters it must be spiritually free also. Food must be simple and pure. It is not possible, according to Krishnamurti, to eat dead animals and be free within oneself. To eat animals means the slavery of those animals. Krishnamurti, in his teachings, therefore takes the standpoint of supporting the whole-food vegetarian, and a Zen Buddhist approach to the spirit and to the emotional is similar to many of the humanist psychologists. In order to be free, one must live in the here and now and reflect the past.

All of these teachings parallel, to some degree, the teachings and philosophy of Acupuncture. They all look for the harmony within the organism, a coming-together of natural forces to produce homoeostasis—internal love, peace and freedom, which will produce external love, peace and freedom—caring. That is health, nothing less. To my mind, this is the true spirit of Acupuncture and of all the vital therapies.

The Acupuncturist, in the old days, looked after the healthy. He was paid to keep his patient fit, and not paid when he was unwell. In ancient China, the patient was responsible for keeping his body supple and beautiful, by exercising and eating pure food, and I believe that this meant vegetarian whole-food.

Further, in his search for harmonious health, the ancient Chinese would look after the emotions. This fact can be gleaned from the Chinese philosophy on how to control the emotions, a discipline in my opinion never to have been bettered. The most successful modern systems are based upon ancient Zen, including Krishnamurti, Gestalt therapy and most of the other humanist psychologies. The control and harmony of the spiritual being follows from a balanced emotional state. In fact, of course, none of the three states could be balanced without the other two. It is all or none.

To consider that Acupuncture can be explained in pure physical terms would turn us away from all the ancient Chinese teachings and thus from the spirit of Acupuncture. It would put us into the realm of modern materialistic western medicine, back into the very area from which so many doctors wish to be freed, the area which is losing the battle against disease, not maybe so much in the physical sense, but in the emotional and spiritual sense. Treating the physical without due consideration to the mental and spiritual is anti-life: only the treatment of the whole being is pro-life.

Acupuncture is essentially a whole-life approach to health and to disease. When talking of Acupuncture, there is never any question of thinking in terms of chemo-therapy, or in terms of molecules, because it is entirely concerned with the spiritual-emotional energy within the organism, which in turn influences the physical. Its very simplicity is its strength.

We now have the opportunity. This is where all the non-orthodox therapists are looking towards us, this is why we have a great responsibility, why we have to blaze the trail towards wholeness in its every form for the west. We must not let down our thousands of colleagues who have been fighting to develop their therapies. We are now rising together. We need each other in our upward surge.

Let us always think in terms of the Acupuncture energy link. This does not mean that chemical constituents and the nervous systems are not involved in acupuncture healing, but that the over-riding principles which control Acupuncture are the principles relating to energy.

Let us keep to our true philosophy and not be side-tracked into the molecular level of western science. Acupuncture can never be explained by nerves, blood, tissue, cells or molecules.

6 Energy Researches

No medicine cures old age or a withered flower — CHINESE PROVERB

RECENT RESEARCHES into the scientific verification of Acupuncture have been far-reaching, and can leave no doubt that the practice is justifiable in terms of Western methods.

The world-wide interest in acupuncture anaesthesia has brought forward many ideas to explain this almost unbelievable phenomenon. When one considers how many other unusual methods of healing exist, it becomes apparent that most of them are ignored by orthodox medicine. It is when confronted with a situation from which there is no escape that explanations begin to emerge.

Healing with the use of magnets has been most successful, but Western science has not been persuaded by this to investigate in any depth. The same applies to faith healing, and who could dare say that faith-healing does not work? Dowsing has been used for many years, either with a pendulum or electro-magnetic instruments, and produces startling results.

Homoeopathy goes back over a hundred years, and the Royal Family always has a homoeopath on its medical staff. In France, almost every other pharmacist is a homoeopathic chemist, and yet Western science makes no scientific evaluation. The followers of Reich have for many years made claims for the success of orgone therapy, and yet the work is mainly underground because of the medical hostility.

Psychic surgery is one of the strangest and most fascinating phenomena in medicine, where actual operations are performed, sometimes without even the use of a knife, and in cases where knives are used, without any sepsis arising, even with the most disreputable tools. Cancers are removed and the patient recovers. (The psychic surgeon believes that the patient is protected by an etheric aura, and that he operates on the living body while protected by the auras.)

Now Acupuncture presents a puzzle to Western medicine which cannot be ignored. It defies all the laws of known medicine. It should not exist; it should not work. If only it could be ignored, like all the other non-orthodox therapies. But it cannot be ignored and it does work, and therefore theories about its mode of action must be produced.

Theories presented by Western scientists require that Acupuncture be fitted into the body of knowledge held by orthodox medicine for, without this, it would remain a mystery.

To postulate a new and hitherto unknown physiological system would be heresy, undermining present thought, leading to the need for a revolutionary re-appraisal of Western concepts of health and disease.

Some Western researchers say, as previously discussed, that acupuncture anaesthesia works by the *gate theory*. According to this theory[15], sensations pass along the peripheral nerve fibres and from there come to what is described as a gate in the spinal cord.

The sensation is allowed to pass through the gate and is then transferred upwards to the brain. In order to experience pain, the gate must be kept open. This is affected by relatively thin fibres which cause the feeling of pain.

The rotating needle in acupuncture anaesthesia is supposed to produce the vibratory effect on the thick fibres and thereby over-ride these thin fibres. The gate locks and stops the transmission to the brain of the pain sensation.

This theory could explain how nerve fibres could be blocked when travelling along the peripheral nerve fibres to the brain via the spinal cord, but it does not explain how abdominal surgery can be performed after needles are inserted in the face, nor how dental extractions can be carried out after the needles are inserted in the arm.

Other researches have presented the proposition that Acupuncture works by hypnosis. By taking this viewpoint, one mysterious form of medicine is being replaced by another, and certainly takes us no nearer to knowing how Acupuncture works, since no-one knows how hypnosis works. Further, the hypnotist himself is by no means happy to be given credit for

15.   Wall, Professor Pat. *New Scientist* 20th July, 1972.

Acupuncture success. Peter Blythe, former Senior Lecturer on hypnosis at Chorley College, has made an extensive study of the subject, and is convinced that there is no hypnotic influence at work. In any case, the hypnosis theory is simple to demolish, because Acupuncture is effective when used on children, even at a very early age "from very young babies to people over eighty"[23].

Another theory as to how Acupuncture works is that it has a placebo effect, and that between forty and seventy per cent of patients would get better whether or not they had any treatment. *Which*[24] conducted a survey on Acupuncture, and investigated exhaustively 232 patients who had had acupuncture treatment, and found that about seventy per cent improved. Considering that three-quarters of these patients had formerly been under conventional drug therapy *without effect,* such results seemed startling, yet the conclusions drawn by *Which* did not reflect this.

In fact, neither the placebo nor the hypnotic effect could be substantiated, in view of the fact that Acupuncture is used effectively on animals. In China, an anaesthetist[25] quotes an experiment wherein animals were bled, to produce a state of intense shock. The one which had been also treated with Acupuncture lived, whereas the untreated one died.

Urquart[26] has stated that there is a rise in the red blood count after acupuncture treatment. Manaka and Tani[27] discovered that, with acupuncture treatment, there are changes in the electro-magnetic field of the body. The experimenters found that pain could be reduced by connecting two metals, copper and zinc, on essential points on the meridians, in a regular order. When the contacts are reversed, the effect is nullified. The treatment followed the ancient rules of Acupuncture, concerning the Yin and the Yang meridians, the Yin being the negative, and the Yang the positive meridian. When the positive impulse is applied to the negative meridian, the pain is relieved, and vice versa, but if like poles are supplied, then pain is not relieved.

23. *Acupuncture Anaesthesia*. Foreign Language Press, Peking 1972. Page 26.
24. *Which* Magazine, London 1972.
25. *Irish Medical Times* 16th June, 1972.
26. Manaka and Urquart. *The Layman's Guide to Acupuncture*. 1972. Page 26.
27. Manaka and Tani. *Electrical Studies on the Skin Surface of the Human Body*. Odswara, Japan. October 1969.

Adamenko[28] has experimented with patients under hypnosis, and discovered that there is a relationship between the energy release at the acupuncture points and the depths of hypnotic trance.

Many researchers have been of the opinion that there must be a connection between the various therapies, which involve the tapping of energy from a common force. These would include Acupuncture, homoeopathy, radionics, spirit and faith healing, magnetic healing and others.

The Russians have been perfecting apparatus to measure these various radiations. One of their first developments is the *tobiscope*[29], which is a machine similar to the kind in use throughout Europe for over twenty years, except that it operates on slightly different principles. The machine has a probe which causes a light to flash when it is over an acupuncture point. This shows that there is increased conductivity over the acupuncture points, a fact which has been demonstrated for many years with the various types of electro-acupuncture apparatus.

The difference between the tobiscope and the more usual pieces of apparatus already in use is that there are no separate positive and negative electrodes. The patient does not hold a negative probe while the operator uses the positive probe. The tobiscope is shaped like a fat pen, pointed at one end. Similar apparatus has been developed separately, in England, by two researchers, Thompson and Gilhead[30].

The tobiscope has the advantage of showing a dim light where there is restricted energy, and differentiating with a bright light, indicating good health at the meridian point. (Most of the latest more-sophisticated acupuncture machines with built-in amp. meters can also distinguish between robust and diminished energy.)

With the development of the tobiscope by Adamenko, the Russians put forward the concept of "bioplasma"[31] as a key to the understanding of the concept of organic energy interaction. The Russians are of the opinion that this organic energy is a fourth dimension, able to transform into other states of matter by certain interactions, just as solids change to liquids and gases.

28.   *Journal of Paraphysics* Volume 6 No. 2 1972. Downtown, Wiltshire: England. Page 82.
29.   Ostrander and Schroeder. *Psychic Discoveries behind the Iron Curtain*, Page 229.
30.   Walter Thompson and Peter Gilhead. Members of the British Acupuncture Association.
31.   Ostrander and Schroeder. Ibid. Many references.

This concept is only a step away from the concept of energy metabolism, whereby plants transform inorganic energy into organic energy, which is then available for animal metabolism. Adamenko believed that it is this *bioplasma,* which explains the workings of Acupuncture.

It is postulated that it is bioplasma which enables a telepathic subject to receive messages from a distance, and others to move objects from a distance. It is bioplasma which is the energy force in radionics, in homoeopathy, in magnetic healing, and it is this force which is being photographed in Kirlian Photography.

Dr. Sergeyev[32], of Russia, has developed the *Piezoelectric Detector of Bioplasm.* The recorder is sensitive enough to register physiological function in every area of the body. The researchers postulate that the electric activity of excited animal cells is actually vibrating low temperature plasma. These investigations led the scientists to believe that this biological plasma (specific organic energy forms) is subjected to exact requirements demanded by thermo-dynamic systems. It was established that vibratory energy levels given off by bioplasma are equal to 7.9 Herz, and equal to the mean frequency intensity fluctuation levels of the earth's magnetic fields.

The totality effect of the living organism results in the emission of concentrated streams of protons and electrons, which then alter the immediate properties of the atmospheric conductivity. From the experiments performed, it was concluded that the atmospheric energy conductivity was altered by the human energy plasma between preset condenser plates. The condenser plates can be set at any distance from the body.

The experiments showed that the greatest amount of bio-plasma energy radiations was concentrated around the cerebral cortex. These microelectro-static charges decrease as the condensers are moved away from the cerebral cortex. The current at the occiput is thirty times as strong as that at the forehead. This fluctuating electro-static emission can concentrate sufficient power to be able to shift an object weighing up to thirty grams in space.

There can be little doubt that a great deal of research will go into determining the power at the acupuncture point, and emissions therefrom, and

32.   Sergeyev Shushkev and Gryaznukkir. *Journal of Paraphysics* Volume 6 No. 1 1972.

into distinguishing it from other animal emissions, in quality and in quantity.

For many years, researches have been going on in naturopathic circles in Germany, into the use of apparatus which can receive and assess signals from various body organs. From these radiations, it can be determined whether the organ is healthy, diseased, or in a pre-disease condition. It is apparent that these many investigations run side by side, and it will not be long before not only will signals from different body areas and organs be plotted, but also the acupuncture points and meridians, according to their intensity and wave length.

Adamenko[28] made a significant advance, and produced a machine to plot the conductivity of the actual meridian channels. This machine uses a combination of points, to make an assessment of the bioplasmic force in the organism. Changes in the energy can be drawn and compared. In one study, a group of volunteers were hypnotised, and mental messages were sent to the hypnotised subjects, from a distant room. The subjects were asked to attempt to pick up the messages, in other words, to use extra-sensory perception. There were definite changes recorded on the instruments, showing that the telepathic messages altered the bioplasmic energy in the subject's organism via the acupuncture meridians. It is, therefore, a distinct possibility that E.S.P. operates via the meridian system.

Some research workers in Russia think that it will be possible to develop human psychic ability, via acupuncture on special points. It appears from the Russian researches that the telepathic messages are picked up, but, because we are not tuned in, the messages never reach the brain. The Russians have been researching with acupuncture points on the arm, which they claim heighten psychic awareness.

In 1939, Davidovich Kirlian[33], an electronic engineer, became interested in high-frequency medical apparatus, after being called in to do a repair. He noticed a flash of light between the electrode and the patient, and wondered what would happen if he placed a photographic plate between the patient and the electrode. Thus was born one of the most fascinating areas of modern scientific discovery, *Kirlian photography.*

28.   *Journal of Paraphysics.* Volume 6 No. 2. Page 82. 1972.

33.   Ostrander and Schroeder. *Psychic Discoveries behind the Iron Curtain.* Page 202.

Kozyrev[34], also in Russia, has developed a new conception of time and space. He postulates that time is denser near the receiver of an action, and thinner near the sender[35].

He has produced experiments to substantiate these theories, with gyroscopes, asymmetrical pendulums and torsion balances. In a simple experiment, a piece of elastic is stretched. It has two poles, the pole at the pull, the causative factor, and the pole at the stretch, or the affected factor. When the elastic is stretched, the measuring instrument, an asymmetrical pendulum made with a gyroscope, is found to arc towards the receiving end, or the stretch or affected end, of the elastic.

This, according to Kozyrev, proves that there is an increase in the density of time at the receiving end. He claims that it is not known energy, as every precaution was taken to shield out electrostatic forces. The experiments have been repeated in different ways, and indicate that chemical reactions act on the arcing of the pendulum, even from a distance.

Kozyrev further claims that emotional thought has a greater influence than intellectual thought, and is convinced that thought changes time-density. He believes that time density can explain how telepathy works, time being thin at the sender's end, and dense at the receiver's end. The balance will be, therefore, to the benefit of the receiver.

Many factors affect time-density, such as the density of matter, the stress which matter is under, the gravitational pull of the earth, electro-magnetic forces, bioplasma, etc. Dr. Kozyrev concerned himself with the fact that everything in nature is asymmetrical, down to the smallest piece of protoplasm.

Kozyrev decided that these spiral circuits were a design of nature, evolved to increase and control energy. (Reich[36] had postulated a similar theory some years earlier). Kozyrev has, further, shown that time is in a positive state, in a left-hand rotating system, and negative, in a right-hand rotating system, and that matter is expanding left-handed positive spiral energy time forms.

34.   Kozyrev, Nikolai *An Unexplored World* Soviet Life. November 1965.
35.   Kozyrev, Nikolai *Possibility of Experimental Study of the Properties of Time.*
      Joint Publications, Research Service, Department of Commerce, U.S.A. 6th May 1968.
36.   Reich, Wilhelm *Cosmic Superimposition.* Orgone Institute Press, Maine, U.S.A. 1951.

This theory ties in perfectly with acupuncture thinking, that energy can be stimulated or sedated, according to the manner in which the acupuncture needle is manipulated — stimulating, when it is excited in a clockwise direction, the bodily effect being a mirror-image of these manipulations, precisely agreeing with the researches of Kozyrev.

7　The Metabolism of Ch'i

The superior doctor prevents illness: the mediocre doctor cures imminent illness: the inferior doctor treats actual illness —

CHINESE PROVERB

IT IS MY CONTENTION that Acupuncture works on the life-force, and not on the body's chemistry. From pure chemical constituents to pure energy, there are many stages. It was once thought that the atom (the smallest single unit of chemistry known to be complete in itself) was solid. Then, it was discovered that the atom itself was composed of many particles; the electrons, neutrons, positrons and other parts are not solid, but are each, in their turn, little universes composed of many parts. It is now postulated that even these particles may not be solid, and so on *ad infinitum*.

But, however minute, there are still particles — particles, and not fields. Pure energy is the *absence* of particles, a wave-form, a field, having *no* mass and *no* form. Energy, by definition, must have no resistance, within or without itself. With no mass, no weight, no form, and no resistance; it must occupy all space for all time, instantaneously. Without form, mass, weight or resistance, it can have no beginning, no end — *no back or front,* as the Chinese would say, occupying all space; it must, at the same time, equate to the occupation of no space.

Because there is no resistance to movement, the energy moves at ultimate speed, yet at no speed. It is absolute movement, and, at the same time, it is still. In its occupation of all space, it occupies no space. Having no weight, it is beyond the conception of weight; having no mass, it is beyond the concept of mass.

Energy is, at one and the same time, Yin and Yang, and yet the absence of yin and yang. Yin and yang is the essence of everything in the universe. Everything has some yin and some yang. Everything is in opposition, and yet complementary. From yin and yang, everything is born. All yin and all yang, in the accepted sense, is found in chemical forms. All chemical forms are in opposition, and complementary, and yet balanced: the atom, the molecule, the unicellular organism, the multi-cellular organism.

Pre-chemical forms are pre-yin and pre-yang, the mother of yin and yang. Energy is the mother of chemistry; chemistry is an expression of yin and yang. Energy, therefore, is also the mother of yin and yang.

Energy must be in a state of balance, and is, therefore, both yin and yang. Being both, it is all, and being all, it is neither. Energy has no back or front, no start or finish, no speed yet all speed, no size yet all size. Energy is the true mother of yin and yang, and, therefore, the true mother of all chemistry.

In Zen philosophy, we see this expressed in many ways, as in meditation, where we seek awareness, and enter into the world of the spiritual, the world of the life force, the life-energy. As we search into our inner self, and live in the here and now, more and more of the Zen concepts become meaningful.

Listening to the sound of the *one hand clapping;* he, who seeks the way, will not find it; the way is here within one; always the zen koan teaches us that, to seek the largest, look at the smallest; to seek the hardest, look at the softest – nothing is softer than water, yet it will wear down the hardest stone. To see the universe, look at the atom. For the bigger yin, look for the bigger yang.

The greater the joy, the greater the possibility of sadness. The more one has, the greater the fear of losing it. The more you have, the more you feel you can lose. What can a man lose, if he has nothing? A man at the bottom can only go up, and a man at the top can only go down.

We can see how Zen interweaves into energy concepts, even although it is thousands of years old. Zen is the philosophical concept of Ch'i, expressed in terms of human meditation. It is the understanding of energy concepts, so far as our spiritual being is concerned.

What lies between energy and matter? Energy is the mother of matter, the mother of yin and yang. Matter, as yin and yang, originates from energy. If matter originates from energy, there must be states of transformation. A coming and going, a form of yin and yang from energy to matter, and a return from matter to energy.

There may, in fact, be hundreds of different stages of energy, between pure energy and matter. It is not possible for Acupuncture to work on true energy, for energy is massless, weightless, shapeless. How, then, can any material form influence energy? Ways have to exist, possibly through a form of bridging arrangement, through which matter and energy can move either way. The bridge represents something which is neither true matter nor true energy.

These *energy-matter-bridges* may be such forces as static electricity, electro-magnetic waves, magnetism, and the life-energy forces. I believe that it is on this level that Acupuncture works.

To illustrate this concept further, I would like to consider certain aspects of food. All food for the animal kingdom comes from the earth. If an animal is a meat eater, unless it is a scavenger, almost without exception, it eats vegetarian animals. Meat-eating animals rarely keep more than one step 'eating-wise' from plant life. Why? I believe the life-energy forces are prepared by the plants, utilising the sun.

The elements needed to sustain life are found in the soil, yet animals cannot live from the soil. It is the plant which takes these elements, and, together with the sun's forces, prepares the food for the animals.

Only at that point can the animal make use of the food, and, with it, the Ch'i synthesized by the plant. The plant food has to be replenished with further plant food, and each meal the animal eats, has to originate from plant food. The vegetarian animal cannot have one meal of plant food, then live directly from the earth.

The meat-eating animal keeps coming back to the vegetarian animal. So that, in the ultimate, every animal lives from plants, and plants live from the earth.

Assuming all the elements the animal needs are contained in the earth, there must be another factor which is needed by the animal, which could be the Ch'i, the life force, our *pre-matter, post-energy* element. Were our assumption to be true, why is the Ch'i consistently needed? There seems to be only one explanation, and that is that the Ch'i is not a catalyst, but has to be metabolized. If it were possible to hold on to the Ch'i, it should be possible to have one meal of plant life, and then many meals of earth.

By thinking along these lines, we can see what is meant by the *vital* force, and why it is found in food, and why food needs to be organic. Chemicals added to the earth, if inert, will tend to damage the Ch'i. The Ch'i, the life-force, is found in the *fruit* of the plant, which holds the seed, and in the *germ* of the cereal. The most vital part of the plant will contain the most Ch'i, and is, therefore, the most health-giving part of the food.

As far as man is concerned, whole-food is healthy food, and is pro-life. The nearer it is to its natural state, the more Ch'i is available. Conversely, the more adulterated the food, the more anti-life it becomes, the Ch'i being damaged, and at a low ebb.

The Ch'i is metabolized, metabolism being a form of yin and yang katabolism and anabolism. The Ch'i is used, and afterwards, there is waste. Everything which lives produces waste. As it is with the chemical part of food, so it must be with Ch'i, the life-energy force.

Solid particles are excreted via the bowels, liquids via the urinary tract, salts via the skin, and gases via the lungs. Where is metabolized Ch'i waste excreted? Could it be through the acupuncture points?

We must, then, consider the possibility that metabolized animal Ch'i is transformed once more, with the help of sunlight, into a new form, to be picked up and utilized by plants, to start a new cycle – a *Ch'i cycle,* as with the nitrogen cycle. Plant Ch'i could then come from the earth elements, or from such a form of Ch'i cycle, or both.

Animals come together with plants, each living on each other, and each producing various cyclic organizations: the nitrogen cycle, the oxygenation cycle, the transpiration cycle, perhaps the Ch'i cycle.

We live and depend upon each other, animals on plants, plants on animals, all depend on the sun, and on the cosmos. Nothing independent, and all are inter-dependent.

It is a simple step to postulate why it is healthier for an animal, if possible, to be vegetarian, for the vegetarian animal is closer the plant Ch'i. When an animal eats another animal, it is eating a metabolized Ch'i, which is toxic and about to be discarded by the other animal. The consuming animal has to handle the toxic Ch'i, and recycle it through its own bodily processes. Perhaps this is why most carniverous animals eat only vegetarian

64

animals, keeping close to the plant Ch'i, and consuming the least amount of toxic metabolized Ch'i. This may be the reason why meat and fish decay, whereas fruit ferments, partly due to the toxic Ch'i.

I have always believed that the experimentation carried out by Professor Kim Bong Han[37] is correct, and will be ultimately accepted. It makes sense to me that the surface meridian network is but the outer layer of an almost infinite number contained in a comprehensive network. Bong Han's theories fit well into my own, and the surface meridian network could well be the channels used to discharge metabolized Ch'i.

Ch'i, being a form of prana, may not be of one form only. Our breathing may bring into our being another form, an electro-magnetic Ch'i. We can influence Ch'i by deep abdominal diaphragmatic breathing, almost certainly, and thus increase our life-energy.

The yogic Ch'i, the Zen Ch'i, the Ch'i we bring in with our breathing, may be concerned with the spiritual being, a spiritual Ch'i; both these forms, and others, being used by the body, the waste eliminated via the acupuncture points. (It seems logical that this form of Ch'i, once used, should undergo similar transformation as the plant Ch'i, and be eliminated via the acupuncture points after use.)

Acupuncture techniques can then be used, if needed, to regulate the Ch'i discharge, either increasing or decreasing as necessary, regulating the internal balance of the various types of Ch'i.

Further, it may even be that the different meridians deal with different forms of Ch'i, some being concerned with plant Ch'i, and others with spiritual Ch'i.

37.   Bong Han Professor Kim *On the Kyungrak System.* Pyongyang, Korea 1964.

8   Orientation Three

It is premature to reduce the vital process to the quite insufficiently developed conceptions of the nineteenth and even twentieth century physics and chemistry — L. DE BROGLIE

AT THIS STAGE. it would be useful to define health, and how Acupuncture fits into the picture.

Health is not just the absence of disease. It is rather a feeling of conscious well-being, something which many people never experience in their entire lives.

It is a physical feeling, a mental-emotional-psychological feeling, and a spiritual feeling — a total expression of the life-forces within the organism.

I want to examine the three prongs of human-ness, the physical, the emotional and the spiritual, and I wish to present the argument that Acupuncture operates through the spiritual (life-energy) into the physical and emotional, as necessary.

Orthodox medicine works mainly on the physical, suppressing or masking symptoms, with apparent improvement to health. In fact, the drugs, being chemically produced and, therefore inert, dampen the activity of the life-force, the vital healing element necessary to all living life-force structures.

Even when orthodox medicine is used on the emotional level, suppressive techniques are used. The drugs employed to treat depression and psychological disorders merely mask the real condition, and, as a result, often the patients become addicted to drugs prescribed for them.

Unfortunately, orthodox medicine not only fails to work through the life-energy forces, but too often, does not even admit to their existence, in the way that the vitalist professions do.

It is my contention that, whereas Acupuncture works through manipulating the life-force energies, and, through them, influences the physical and the mental, orthodox medicine works almost exclusively on the chemical and the atomic structure of the physical being, using methods which merely conceal the symptoms, instead of recognizing and using them as *Nature's early warning system.*

If the symptoms were the disease, then it would be logical to suppress them. But is the phlegm of a cold, the cold? No. Is it then logical to stop the mucous escaping? Is a fever the disease? No. Is it then logical to stop the fever? Or, only to control it? The rubbish we expel in bronchitis, is it the disease? No. Why, then, should we attempt to stop the elimination of the mucous? Is pain itself a disease? No. Should we, therefore, just prevent the person from feeling the pain?

The case for symptom treatment is not justified. The more potent and advanced the drugs become, the more they mask the real cause of disease; the more they restrict the organism from using its own recuperative powers, building up its own inner reserves.

Pain control is one field in which there are great dangers for the Acupuncturists, for high precision, suppressive techniques have been developed. Already, one has only to look at the pain-control institute of Japan[38] to see a whole international organization devoted exclusively to methods of pain control, which, in turn, mean suppression, and, mainly by the use of Acupuncture; to my mind, a misapplication.

As far as we are aware, the traditional Chinese doctor did not use Acupuncture as a panacea, but, even if he had, it is not up to us to follow blindly. We must develop our own judgements, in the light of our own experience and understanding. Personally, I am convinced that it is the life-force which is the most important function in the organism, not the physical or the mental, once more taking us back to the logic of the vital energy.

In my opinion, Acupuncture works, not only on the level of the life-force, but influences the physical and the mental, by bringing to them life-energy, thereby stimulating and increasing their resistance, and bringing into use all the inherent powers within the organism.

Each organism functions as an integrated whole, with each part functioning as a unit within this integrated whole. Within a body, the circulatory system functions, the liver functions, the heart functions, each according to its own pattern.

38.   The Kioto Pain Control Institute, 280 Shimizucho Takatsuji Kawaramachi,
       Shimogyo, Kyoto, Japan.

There is an organic and a systemic build-up of cellular structure (which comes from food). The body knows when to make brain cells, when to make muscle cells—how to make them, where to make them, how many to make, where to put them, how to dispose of them.

All this is related to the overall body functional integrity of an infinite number of functions, which, to my mind, has to be related to the life-force, whatever that may be. It cannot be related to body chemistry, because chemistry begins and ends with the ectoderm of the atom. So, logic tells us that energy outside the atom must exist. Except through an energy form, how could atoms communicate? If energy outside the atom were not to exist, there could be no communication between atoms, there could be no structural integration, no integrated function within the organism.

The body is a functioning integrated unit, with the instinct that, if necessary, for the good of the whole, a part may be sacrificed.

Vital medicine is related to the life-force, and it is on this level that acupuncture works. Acupuncture does not work because it systematically stimulates the nerve cells. If acupuncture treatment stimulates nerve cells, it is because, at that moment, the body's inherent life-force needs to use nerve impulses. At other times, it will use the hormonal system, the endocrinal system, the glandular or the circulatory system, or even further systems of which we are as yet unaware.

Attempting to isolate a part from the whole teaches us little or nothing. It is possible for a part to function in isolation temporarily, such as a heart continuing to beat. But will it renew its own cells? Will it renew itself? Everything in the body *functions*, and it is the function that counts. Microscope work can only explain structure, never function. Orthodox medicine works in attempting to control structure artificially with drugs, but in the process, the function becomes damaged, because, in Nature, it is function which controls structure, through a process of priority, working from the more important to the less important, so that, when structure is interfered with, function will be disturbed. This is why the drug approach cannot, in the long run, cure disease.

Further, the disturbance of already damaged structure disturbs the life-force, which should be controlling the function, and this, in turn, disturbs both function and structure.

Apart from the life-force, the physical structure depends on nutrition and movement. Movement means work, exercise. Incorrect movement will result in disease, because the body structure is not nourished correctly.

The best exercises are those which bring into play the physical, the mental and the spiritual. (The spiritual is the life-force on a conscious level.) The best exercises are, therefore, walking, running, yoga, the martial arts such as judo; as, between them, they bring into use the three aspects of life.

Behind all good exercise lies the correct use of the diaphragm. Here, the body, with deep breathing, gets into touch with the source of its well-being, its life-energy. The yogis have always known this, and tell us that the breath of life enters the body through the navel, and replenishes the life-force.

Through body tensions, we use the diaphragm less, and, as we get older, by the time we are about forty years of age, we hardly use it at all, becoming upper respiratory breathers. The diaphragm is *Nature's masseur*, massaging the abdominal and the thoracic organs, and helping the structural integrity of the organisms, life-energy. Correct breathing, through the diaphragm, increases the life span, by not only sufficiently oxygenating the body, but by drawing in ample life-energy.

Tension shortens the spine, the contracting muscles collapse the spring-like structure of the spinal column, and, consequently, the life-force, which works very closely with our nervous system, is disturbed. We are as integral a part of the air we breathe as the heart is a part of the body. We can only live for minutes without air. Equally, we are a part of the sun, for, without the sun, nothing would grow, and the world would decay. We need sunlight; it nourishes the life-force, maybe even builds it. There is much sense in the worship of a sun-God. When we lie in the sun, we can feel the life energy flowing, being nourished.

There are techniques which can be developed for getting in touch with this life-force — through meditation, judo. It is what we use in intuition, E.S.P., healing, in love, in compassion. Birds use it. It is within us, available at all times. When we feel compelled to do something out of love or compassion, when a feeling comes over us, which is beyond us, and we act without conscious thought, we are in contact with it. It comes to us when we just *know* something, something that we cannot explain, a flash of intuition.

70

Under these conditions, we are using the universal intelligence, the life-force, the etheric force, the prana, the Ch'i, tapping into the universal nirvana, slipping into The Way, for a brief moment. We all use it, but, by not recognizing it, by refusing to acknowledge it, we lose much of our ability to utilize these forces for our own integrated health, and for the good of others.

Clean air, sunlight, life-energy exercises are all pro-life. Toxic air, lack of exercise, lack of sun, incorrect breathing are all anti-life.

Food, when adulterated, becomes less pro-life. The more it is processed and chemicalized, the more it becomes 'plastic' food and anti-life. Anti-life food moves the organism towards disease. The more the food is changed from its *ground-found* form, the more it is disturbed in the ground by chemicals, then the more the life-energy which exists within food, is disturbed.

As food is needed for life, is it not logical to assume that the life-energy forms in the food are related to our own life-energy forms? Our energy patterns are disturbed, and we move towards disease. Disturb the plant-energy patterns, and our own energy patterns are disturbed, and we move towards disease. *Disease is an attempt on the part of the body to regain health,* by bringing attention to the anti-life actions which have been taken against the organism.

Whole-food is full of life-energy; not devitalized food, nor tinned, fried, adulterated, sprayed, insecticided, herbicided, separated or frozen foods. Whole-food includes roughage, bran, germ, the whole organism, with its vitamins, trace elements, minerals, plus a myriad of unknown vital factors. It should be prepared with love, for, through love, we express life-energy patterns, and harmonize them with the very food presented.

By nature, man is a vegetarian animal, taking his life-energy forms direct, not via the animal's metabolized (Ch'i) energy, which is toxic.

Life-force is subtle, soft, gentle and easily disturbed, and needs to be handled with tenderness and care. Appropriate, therefore, is Acupuncture as a form of medicine, as it is subtle, tender and caring. Acupuncture treatment moves gently into the life-energy patterns of the patient.

The physical side of health is only one part of the triangle, and the emotional and spiritual are of great importance. Who would postulate which is the most important? I do not wish to spend time discussing the emotional side of health, as there are excellent methods available to restore mental balance. Here again, orthodox medicine, with its obsession with drugs, has failed, and it is the new therapies which are having the successes. Jung, Freud, Adler and others did a new and interesting job in medicine, but the time was not then ripe for the coming break-through. Reich, alas, was also before his time, and the American orthodox scene hit him hard; but his work lives on and grows.

Soon after the war, Scientology came on to the scene, a form of westernized Zen. In spite of some dangers in Scientology through it becoming a personality cult, thousands of people have been helped.

But it was in the 1960's that the real break-through began: Gestalt, relaxation, meditation, bio-energetics, co-counselling, encounter, biofeedback, psycho-drama, psycho-synthesis — the humanist psychologies were born.

New giants of thought became known, who really could point the way to help people's emotional problems; Krishnamurti, Carl Rogers, Maslow, Illich, Barry Stevens, Orgage, Gurdjieff, Reich, Assagioli, Laing, Watts, Ouspensky, Janov and a host of others. These new therapies, loosely linked together under the title of the *humanist psychologies,* were not suppressive. They encouraged people to find freedom within themselves.

They all accept Acupuncture, for they see in it something akin to what they are doing themselves.

We are seeking a way of directing man's inner forces, his life's energy, his Ch'i. We are not suppressing, and our work is pro-life. The humanistic psychologists are our new-found allies, more so even than the traditional naturopath, osteopath and chiropractor.

The final side of our triangle is the spiritual, the life-force. It is the use of intuition, E.S.P., our energy-forces, feeling them, contacting them. It is not easy to say where the spiritual, the life-energy patterns begin, and where the emotional, the mental, the psychological, end. They interweave endlessly. Religious people think of the spiritual in terms of God, the soul, while non-religious people think in terms of life-energy.

Life-energy patterns, life forms, undoubtedly exist. With Acupuncture, we influence these life-energy forms. We contact our energy forces through the physical and the emotional, by meditation, by diaphragmatic breathing, by Acupuncture, by awareness; by recognizing that we are alive now, by being aware of this moment.

The humanist psychologies teach us that life is in the here and now. To live in the past is to live with images. All thought is of the past, and not of reality, as there is no reality of the past. The past is a series of images. From the past, people project into the future; ideals. From the images of the past, we project ideals for the future continually and ceaselessly, living in a dream world, an unreal world, the world of the physical and the emotional. The only reality is the present, the momentary and everlasting here and now. This is the lesson of Zen.

In the here and now is unlimited energy, says Krishnamurti. Images are inner conflicts, and every image steals needed energy. To be free of images and of ideas, is to be free of conflict. To be free of conflict, is to have unlimited energy. To be aware, to be free, to express yourself through your intuition, is to be in constant close touch with the life-force; to feel love of all people, of the plants, the trees, the animals, to have boundless energy. This, then, is health, the completion of the triangle, the physical, the emotional and the spiritual. Then, when all else is in harmony, should there come the slightest disturbance, and a need for re-balancing, there is only one true medicine, which is, of course, Acupuncture.

9 Lakhovsky and Eeman

To seek the largest, look at the smallest — ZEN KOAN

I WOULD LIKE TO LOOK at two attempts by diverse researchers to investigate the mystery of energy and its use for health; namely, Lakhovsky and Eeman. Many of you will be familiar with their works, but a few minutes looking at their achievements, and then attempting to relate them to Acupuncture, can do no harm.

Lakhovsky[39] invented the Multi Wave Oscillator, or M.W.O. He died as recently as 1942, and he did most of his research before the second world war. His theory was that every living thing emits radiations. From this simple premise, he was able to explain almost all phenomena in nature, including E.S.P., migration, health and disease. He maintained that health was enhanced, and, in fact, only possible, when the oscillations were at the exact wave-length related to each organ, structure and cell in the body. Disease was associated only with disharmony in the radiations. Could any Acupuncturist disagree with this conception?

He likened the cell to an *oscillating electric circuit,* each cell vibrating at a specific and set speed and frequency. Lakhovsky claimed that the cell vibrations were controlled and maintained by cosmic interactions. According to his teachings, oscillate and live, *oscillate correctly and live harmoniously.* Oscillating changes cause disharmony and disease. If the oscillation ceases, or slows down too fundamentally, then death ensues. His theories explain why whole-food (brown bread, sugar, rice, etc.) maintains balance, while devitalized foods cause disease. The oscillations have been disturbed.

The body must be fed with correct cellular-cosmic radiations, pulsating in perfect harmony. The atomic parts, the electrons, protons, neutrons and positrons are circumscribed entities, which, by definition, have no life outside their own ectoforce (their limiting outsides). Therefore, the force which makes

39.   Lakhovsky, G. *The Secret of Life.* Heinemann 1933.

them oscillate, must be outside the atom, and associated with energy. This is what I call an *energy bridge,* not pure energy.

Pure energy must be functional, occupying all space instantaneously, with unlimited superimposition one energy upon another. Energy bridge oscillations disturb the function of pure energy, and thereby condense the pure energy, this energy bridge being a form of *non-energy non-matter;* but between them both.

It would appear that Lakhovsky's theory on cell oscillation is a form of energy bridge; a bridge between pure function-energy and matter. It could be that it is on this level that Acupuncture operates, in the field of oscillation, the field of energy-matter-bridging. Lakhovsky produced from a Tesla coil his M.W.O., and, with this machine, he achieved great healing.

It is not my intention to discuss this machine, or Lakhovsky and his work any further, only to show how, as with Reich and Homoeopathy, and other forms of non-orthodox healing, we are again dealing with wave-forms, radiations, oscillations, electro-magnetic waves, the Ch'i of life. We will discover that there are many other methods developed to achieve the same results as Acupuncture, and that there are already many disciplines in existence, which are working along the same lines.

Let us now look at the works of Eeman[40]. He said that "When different parts of one human body, or different or similar parts of different human bodies, are connected by means of an electrical conductor, such as insulated wires, these bodies behave as though, using an electro-magnetic analogy, they were *bi-polar*".

Eeman discovered that the body has both positive and negative poles. The head is positive, and the base of the spine negative. The right hand is positive and the left hand negative, in right-handed people, the converse being true of left-handed people.

Eeman used a simple copper screen with a hand probe. He discovered that, when polar opposites are connected, a relaxation effect is produced, but that, if polar similars are connected, stimulation is produced, very similar to the acupuncture yin-yang principle.

No-one, as yet, has been able to measure the forces at work with the Eeman screen, yet thousands of patients have benefitted from its use. Many blind tests were conducted, to show conclusively that the results were not due to psychological factors.

He found that relaxing circuits fostered better sleep, recovery from fatigue and disease, increased the capacity for work, and improved health generally. The tension circuit reversed these effects, producing discomfort.

Eeman concluded that the nervous system behaved as though there were electro-magnetic opposition between its different parts, in other words a form of oscillation. Here, Eeman and Lakhovsky appear to have been working on the same line, from different viewpoints. It is easy to assume that the Eeman circuit may work on and influence the same forces as used in Acupuncture, the bridges between energy and matter.

The East and the non-orthodox West have not been far apart in their search for health, using different paths, but fundamentally achieving similar results. Probably, many of these methods use what Acupuncturists call *Ch'i*. Before long, we may find that there will be even more methods developed to harmonise the Ch'i. Already, we have Acupuncture itself, moxibustion, Eeman techniques, multi-wave oscillators, homoeopathy, magnets, etc., all working towards harmony and balance.

10 Magnetic Healing

To see the universe, look at the atom — ZEN SAYING

ACUPUNCTURE WORKS by stimulating, organising, sedating, rebalancing the body's electro-magnetic forces. We cannot consider that there is only one form of such force in nature, or in the human organism. There may well be hundreds, if not thousands, of different forms of energy, which the organism utilises, and which come under the influence of acupuncture therapy and prophylaxis. I believe that the body attracts these energy manifestations via two main channels, the food we eat, and the air we breathe.

When speaking in terms of electro-magnetic forces, we find ourselves at a disadvantage, because there is no precise vocabulary to describe such various forces. We have some inadequate words and expressions, such as *magnetism, human magnetism, mesmerism, electro-magnetism, static electrical forces, life force, vital energy, Ch'i, prana, life energy* and a few others. They overlap in meaning, but have never been defined clearly; which is not surprising, as they are non-material forces in Nature, as difficult to explain as it would be to explain how a blade of grass grows.

I re-iterate that I do not believe that it is true energy which is used by plants or animals, but rather a form of post-energy, or pre-matter, for which I have coined the term *'Energy-Bridge'*. Even this is an inadequate term, as it implies only one form of energy, when, I am convinced, there are at least two main forms used by the body, and there could be hundreds.

In looking at magnetic healing, I want to concentrate upon hand therapy — the use of the hands for healing.

My contention is that the life force energy enters the body from the food that we eat, and from the air that we breathe, which we metabolize, use as a form of energy, life-force, and eliminate through the acupuncture pores. Should the energy be dammed up, acupuncture techniques can be used to release and regulate it. In other words, it can normalize a yang condition. If the body is *losing* too much Ch'i, Acupuncture can be used to stimulate and regulate the yin condition towards the yang, and normality. Further, the body must have mechanisms whereby, as it only utilizes the amount of Ch'i it requires, it allows surplus Ch'i to be expelled. For example, surplus Ch'i in the oxygen, might be expelled through exhalation, and superfluous life energy taken in with food, could be eliminated via the bowels.

In normal life, of breathing and feeding, there is sufficient of everything — food, air, life-energy, with plenty to spare. Nature works this way, if possible. Normally, surplus is expelled *before* metabolism. In my opinion, any surplus energy which has been metabolized is controlled by the mechanism of the surface acupuncture points. Therefore, when there is a condition of tension (yang), the acupuncture pores are in tension, and the electro-magnetic pressures are disturbed in such a way that insufficient used life energy is escaping through the pores. Thus, it continues to circulate through the meridian system, through every cell in the body, slowly poisoning the whole organism. This is *yang toxaemia,* manifested in headaches, migraine, high blood pressure.

Conversely, in old age, where there are flaccidity and yin conditions, it is a different picture. In this case, too *much* Ch'i is escaping via the acupuncture pores, and the patient is literally falling away, lacks energy, is always tired, and so on. For this type of condition, Acupuncture is used in a yang way — for, not only is the toxic metabolized energy escaping, but also the body is losing needed life-energy, thereby producing the conditions of yin.

On investigating hand healing, magnetic healing, in the light of this contention, it can be seen that there is always an abundant supply available to the healer. As already explained, I believe that we normally take in a great deal more life energy than we need when we breathe, and we normally expel the surplus.

However, it is possible to learn to retain some of this surplus, to be used for healing. With training, we can develop the ability; and our hands, particularly the tips of the fingers, being the most sensitive parts of our bodies, are where we store it. They are infinitely more sensitive than the most sensitive modern machines. As practitioners of Acupuncture, we are aware of this. Thus, healers are using the *source* of all healing, the surplus life-force. Everyone has the ability to heal latent within them, and all can develop its use.

80

Hippocrates wrote "It hath oft happened, while I have been soothing a patient, as if there were some strange property in my hand, to pull and draw away from the afflicted part aches and divers impurities, by laying my hands on the place and by extending the fingers towards it."

A healer replenishes the energy he gives out. As it leaves his hands, more is drawn in through the lungs. A healer who gets exhausted is not using his healing powers correctly.

It has often been said that healing is psychological, just as it has been said of Acupuncture. But, as with Acupuncture, healing has been consistently and effectively used on animals.

It seems that the energy flow from the hands can be picked up by the patient's body at any point. The best parallel to this, is in terms of high frequency electricity, in a spark produced across a gap. It may well be that the high intensity life-force given off by a trained healer is forced through the skin in the same way. The healer's surplus energy is thus picked up and utilized by the patient.

Being surplus energy, it is always fresh, and in no way toxic, energy. Sometimes, patients are afraid to take part in a healing circle, lest they pick up toxic energies from other patients. If the aforementioned theory is correct, this is not possible, as the energies involved are drawn fresh from the cosmos, thus always new and pure and healing. There is absolutely nothing to fear.

There is even a method whereby the energy emanating from the hands can be seen. Place some black material on a table, dim the lights, and then point the outstretched fingers at each other at a distance of two inches. If the position is kept for about two minutes, to allow the eyes to become accustomed to the light, emanations forming a cobweb pattern can often be seen. If no energy can be seen, then the vitality is low. In that case, if the fingers are brought closer together, the emanations will probably become visible. This is a test of personal vitality, at any given time.

It is also a test to discern if someone will make a good healer. When the energy is high, it is possible to move the fingers further apart, and still see the emanations. A really good healer, in good vitality, will have emanations of about four inches.

The colour of these emanations vary from grey to blue. The more blue, the more vital the person, and the greater the healing power. Most people give off a greyish-blue hue. This test has been taken further by Kilner[41], who describes a method for discerning a patient's health by their overall aura vitality.

The approach used is based upon the above observation, with the patient completely undressed, and the practitioner discerning the vitality. Using magenta glasses, he peers into the daylight for about a minute, then he takes off the glasses, and looks at the patient, who is standing against a dark background, in a darkened room, which enhances the aura effect. The intensity of the blue, the grey or the mixture, and how far the aura spreads out from the body are all noted.

If there is a break anywhere in the outline, it means that there is trouble in the area, for the aura is damaged. (Dr. Kilner discovered that the aura disappeared from the body at death.) Further, it was found that changes could be brought about in the aura, if the subject carried out certain concentration exercises.

Dr Kilner also invented a screen which showed up the utra-violet end of the spectrum. By using this apparatus, Dr. Kilner was able to show the density, shape and texture of the energy aura.

For centuries, clairvoyant people have claimed to see auras. Now machines have been invented so that ordinary people can see them also, just as, in Acupuncture, electro-acupuncture apparatus has been developed to enable the scientist to establish that the meridians exist.

In my opinion, the energy which we have been discussing here, is not physical energy, the energy associated with food, which goes to feed the physical being. It is the energy we obtain from the air we breathe, which goes towards feeding the spiritual being, the life-energy. Again, it must be stressed that the term 'energy' is being loosely used. I prefer to call it a *post-energy pre-matter* energy bridge.

For many years, it has been known that magnetic healing is most effective if the patient lies from north to south, head north and feet south. This fits into the very old theory that one should always sleep with the head to the

41. Kilner, Walter *The Kirlian Aura*. New York. University Books 1965.

north and the feet to the south, in order to magnetize the body, and increase the personal energy.

What has been known for thousands of years in Acupupuncture has its counterpart in the two to three hundreds of years of experience in healing, and also with the work of Eeman. Each group, by its own experiences, has come to a similar conclusion. Kushi[42], perhaps one of the world's authorities on healing, presents similar conclusions, reached after the thousands of years of palm healing practised in Japan.

In a right-handed person, the right hand is positive, yang. In a left-handed person, the *left* hand is positive, yang. In each case, the other hand is, of course, yin. This is very important to remember. When treating by healing, it must be remembered that some form of electro-magnetic force is being used. Just as in a magnet, like poles repel, and opposites attract.

Therefore, to produce a yang effect, the healer would use his yang hand on the yin side of the patient's body, thereby stimulating the yin side with the healer's yang. To produce a yin effect, exactly the reverse approach is used – the healer would use his yin hand on the patient's yang side.

The next point to recognize is that the head is positive, yang, and the base of the spine, negative, yin. This is universal. But, in a right-handed person, the right side of the head will be most positive, yang, slowly becoming less yang towards the centre of the head. The left side of the head will be quite neutral, the left side of the body's yin being neutralized by the head's yang.

The whole of the procedure of the various aspects of yin and yang can be worked out in this respect; the back, being yang, and the front yin. The head yang and back yang is the same for both left-handed and right-handed people, the variation being solely in the right side and the left side. It is, therefore, quite simple to produce a set of working rules as to how to create a yin or a yang effect using magnetic hand healing. Stroking from the head towards the base of the spine is more yin than stroking from the base of the spine towards the head, which is more yang.

The greatest yang effect is created when the treatment is given on the left side of the back, from the base of the spine to the head with the yang

42.   Kushi, Michio. Founder East West Foundation.

hand. The greatest yin effect is produced by treating the patient's spine, by stroking the right side with the yin hand from the head down to the base.

I have not studied spiritual healing, as achieved by healers who simply put their hands on an affected part. However, everyone who does healing will, at times, use the laying on of hands on an affected part, thus allowing the life-force to flow into the patient. The patient will experience all sorts of results; sometimes nothing; feeling nothing, but having good results; tingling; electric shocks; waves; heat; tickly feelings; etc.

During healing, it is always essential that rhythmic diaphragmatic breathing take place. The Hindus claim that the life-force 'prana' is drawn in with the breath; Baron von Reichenbach called it the 'odic' force. We call it *Ch'i*, life-energy, life-force. Yogis, under laboratory conditions, have proved that they happily exist with one breath a minute, whereas the average individual needs twelve. Normally, we only take in about 500 c.c. of air with each breath, whereas it is possible to develop to quadruple this intake, with training. With exercises, it is possible that an experienced Yogi can hold as much as eight to ten litres at any one time. Think of the great amount of surplus vital energy which is available for healing in these conditions. It means that the healer can use the surplus without tiring or exhaustion.

11 Kim Bong Han

There is a principle which is a bar against all argument. That principle is condemnation before investigation — HERBERT SPENCER

KIM BONG HAN[43] has, for a number of years, been questioning the failure of modern medicine and biology to elucidate the mechanisms underlying the unity of the activities of the organism. He looked for a solution in the traditional school of medicine, called the *Kyungrak* system.

Bong Han has shown that there are four series of meridians in the organism. Spaced at intervals along these meridians, or ducts, are small corpuscles, and each duct or meridian may contain scores of ductules, which measure on average from 5-15 microns across, although the range is from one to fifty microns.

The first of the meridian systems is called the *Internal Duct System*. These ducts are found, free floating, in the vascular and lymphatic vessels. The ductules ramify, so that the path of the containing vessels are completely followed.

Flowing in all ductules is a fluid or liquor. In the Internal Duct System, the liquor generally follows the blood or lymph flow, but, in some cases, it runs in the opposite direction. Also, these internal ducts penetrate beyond the vessels. These facts led Bong Han to the conclusion that the formation of the Internal ducts is different in origin from that of the blood and lymph vessels.

The second series of meridians is the *Intra-External Duct* System. These are found on the surface of the internal organs, and they form a network which is entirely independent of the vascular, the lymphatic and the nervous systems.

The third series is the *External Duct* System. These run alongside the outer surface of the walls of the vascular and lymphatic vessels. These ducts are also found in the corium, and are here known as the *Superficial Duct* System. It is this latter system with which we are most familiar in

Acupuncture. The fourth series of ducts is known as the *Neural Duct* System. These are distributed in the central and peripheral nervous systems.

All of the various duct systems are interlinked via the connection of the terminal ductules of the different systems, very much as in the case of the arterioles which link with the venules, bringing together the arteries and veins. Bong Han has shown that myeloid and lymphatic elements exist in the ducts. When erythrocytes in the bone marrow and the peripheral blood system are killed with phenylhydrazine, activity in the corpuscles increases, and they enlarge. By contrast, anaemia develops when the Internal Duct System is injured. This suggests that hematopoiesis is one of the functions of the internal meridians.

To show the control of the meridians over a particular organ, Bong Han severed the portal duct of a frog, and found that histological changes soon took place in the *liver*. The cells enlarged, and the cytoplasm became turbid. Within three days, serious vascular degeneration took place throughout the whole liver. Many other experiments confirmed these results.

Bong Han conducted a series of tests to establish the constituents of the duct liquor. He isolated nearly as much Hyaluronic acid as is found in sperm; twenty different kinds of free amino-acids, including all of the essential ones; sixteen different free mononucleotides, corticosteroid, ketosteroid, oestrogen and adrenalin. Over twice as much adrenalin as discovered in the blood was isolated, and, in an acupuncture point, over ten times as much was found. Bong Han also isolated both desoxyribonucleic acid (D.N.A.) and ribonucleic acid (R.N.A.) from the liquor.

The existence of hyaluronic acid, cortical and medullary hormones and oestrogen suggest that the Kyungrak system is closely associated with the endocrine system. To investigate the liquor flow, Bong Han injected radio isotope Phosphorus 32 (P32) into an acupuncture point. Microautoradiography was possible in two hours in the external corpuscles. No. P32 was detected in the blood vessels. P32, injected into an internal corpuscle, was quickly labelled in the internal ducts, but only slowly found its way to the superficial system. P32, injected into the ear vein could hardly be detected anywhere in the Kyungrak network.

These experiments show that the Kyungrak system is independent of the vascular system; the meridian liquor flows from the acupuncture points inwards, to the deeper ducts and corpuscles, and finally outwards again.

Bong Han has shown that the terminal ductules reach the tissue cell nuclei. P32 injected into ducts found its way to the cell nuclei. Bong Han concluded that, not only is the Kyungrak system interlinked, but that *all* cell nuclei are interwoven into the system. Working on the embryonic chick, Bong Han found that, basically, the Kyungrak ducts were formed within fifteen hours of conception, by which time the primordia of the organs are not yet formed. He suggests that the function of the Kyungrak system exerts an influence upon the differentiation of cells. Further, the positioning of the Kyungrak system in the embryo is completed earlier than any of the other organistic parts.

Having conducted experiments on mammals, aves, reptiles, amphibia, pisces, invertebrates and hydra, Bong Han suggests that the Kyungrak system exists in all multicellular structures, both animal and vegetable.

Unique granules circulate in the duct liquor. These granules have been named *Bong Han Sanal*. The Sanal develops into cells and, after a lapse of time, converts back into sanal. There is a continuous renovation of cell tissue, which is controlled by the Kyungrak system. Sanal contains D.N.A., R.N.A. and protein. Bong Han claims to have been able to grow *in vitro* cells from Sanal.

The concept is that sanal flows in the meridian liquor. It forms by fusion into a cell and, after a limited life, bursts through the cell membrane to recirculate in the ducts as 'sanal'. In the course of the formation of a cell from sanal, the D.N.A. content is increased sixteen times, R.N.A. nine times and protein nitrogen thirty-two times. Besides Bong Han's discovery of cell formation from sanal, he also appears to have made important observations concerning cell division. When the cell is a stable unit, the sanal is in a fused state. During cell division, it breaks down in a way which suggests the behaviour of chromosomes. If the cell is fixed after the nuclear membrane has broken down, the sanal gives every appearance of chromosomes, being the same in number as usually found in the cell of the animal under investigation. Bong Han claims that chromosomes, appearing at cell division are, in fact, sanal and cell division is a specific form of movement of sanal. The inheritance of life attributed to chromosomes is an aspect of sanal, and part of the organization of the meridians.

The cell theory holds that the cell is the uniting morphological and functional unit of the organism, and that cells are formed only from cells through cell division. The Bong Han experiments are inconsistent with this theory. Bong Han used P32 to identify sanal extracted from an acupoint. The extracted sanal was injected into different parts of the circulating ducts. According to Bong Han, within forty-eight hours, tagged sanal could be detected among cell tissues. This experiment suggests that sanal from the corpuscles eventually become part of the tissue cell. These observations were confirmed by many experiments, including those on the ovary, the suprarenal body, the liver, the kidney and the lungs.

Bong Han considered that, as the various acupuncture points have specific connections with relevant bodily organs and functions, then sanal taken from different parts should produce different types of cells. He conducted a series of three hundred and forty-four experiments, taking sanal from seventy-nine different acupoints. As was expected, different cells were formed in accordance with the foci of those points.

Bong Han's final series of experiments (about which we have knowledge) concerns the photo-chemical influence of light in the epidermis. Sanal, cultivated under normal light, grew one hundred and four cells in ninety-six hours, whereas in a dark chamber, only thirty-two were formed. After seventy-two hours in the dark chambers, *no* more new cells were formed. He attributed the few cells which did grow in the dark to having already been under the photo-chemical influence of light in the superficial corpuscles, before being extracted from the ducts. In other words, he claims that cells, at some stage, and in some way, must, during their growth, be charged with "energy" rays, influenced by light.

Since 1970, contact with Bong Han has been lost to the west, and it is not known if his researches are continuing. Several workers have attempted to reproduce his results, with varying results. One or two scientists claim his researches to have been largely or entirely false, while others are saying that his results are demonstrable.

One thing is certain. If only a small part of Bong Han's work should be proved correct, the whole medical chemical philosophy will have to be re-evalutated in the light of hormonal-energy relationships.

12   Acupuncture and Orgone

When one is confronted with a fact which is in opposition to prevalent theory, one must accept the fact, and abandon the theory, even though the latter, supported by great men, may be generally subscribed to. —

CLAUDE BERNARD

BOTH ACUPUNCTURE AND REICH'S CONCEPT of the orgone (OR) are based upon the principle of a life energy. A study of the ways in which each describes the life energy, its flow, and methods of influencing it, would be of interest because of the possibility for a diagnostic and therapeutic relationship between the two. Hopefully, this comparison may lead to therapeutic successes, which are not present in either system alone.

Both systems have achieved increasing recognition in the western world in the past few years. The ideas of Reich are now widely accepted in psychological circles, and used as the basis for different types of therapies, such as bio-energetics, Gestalt, primal therapy, encounter, and various forms of armour break-down massage. The rapidly increasing use of Acupuncture in the western world is also well known.

We will specifically compare the life energies assumed by classical Acupuncture, the "Ch'i", and the "OR" described by Reich, since both descriptions are central to their systems.

Both Ch'i and orgone energy stand outside the framework of prevailing western biology and medicine.

The western traditional ideas are based upon an investigation of life at the molecular level. For such investigation, molecules are isolated from their organisms, placed in an unnatural environment, and then their properties are studied. The idea is to reduce the components of life to their "simple" constituents, attempt to understand functioning at this level, and then to work back, in an attempt to understand the living organism. This method manifestly fails, as we can see by the limited progress achieved, and the vast areas of total failure in orthodox research.

This approach fails to understand the life force, frequently fails to grasp even the function, achieving its main and limited success in *pathology*. The reason is obvious, looked at from a vitalist viewpoint. Orthodox biology and medicine concentrate upon isolating tissues, as in biopsy, and, as the tissue is no longer *in situ*, its function is, perforce, impaired and altered. Thus the investigation is relatively fruitless, so far as understanding function, and quite useless as far as the study of energy is concerned.

Another contrast between the conventional approach on the one hand, and Acupuncture and Reich on the other hand, is in methodology. The conventional method is based upon complete objectification, and the belief that it can ultimately conquer nature, along with a strict dualism between subject and object, whereas Acupuncture and Reich both attempt to harness and co-operate with nature.

It is true that, philosophically, the west talks about the relationship between investigator and subject, based upon the Heisenberg uncertainty principle. But, in practice, in biology and medicine, there is strict separation between the investigator and subject. The Taoist thinking, associated with Acupuncture, does not make sharp divisions between material and non-material, organic and inorganic, living and dead. One *eases* into the other, one comes from the other. According to this thinking, there are two cosmic forces, two energy principles, through and around which everything radiates. These are the complementary principles of Yin and Yang, the negative and the positive. Yin is the negative, receptive, female element, and, in its extreme form, typifies coldness, death and darkness. Yang is the positive, outgoing, male element, and brings forth warmth, vitality and light.

Reich also came to the conclusion that biological energy circulates longitudinally up and down the body. He arrived at this conclusion on the basis of psychiatric observations. In neurotic cases, the resistance to the flow of energy are the blocks, which are roughly perpendicular to the energy flow.

The functional method of thought, which Reich termed his methodology, is essentially the same as used by the ancient Chinese. Reich[44] notes the similarity between his functionalism and Chinese early thinking.

44.   Reich, Wilhelm *Ether, God and Devil.* Orgone Institute Press, Maine, U.S.A. 1949.

This similarity he attributed to the fact that early thinking was not yet bogged down in detail.

The location of the acupuncture meridians may be taken as a systematized description of the flow described by Reich.

Let us compare the direction of the energy flow, as described by Acupuncture and Reich[45], who compares the human with the worm, and states that the flow of energy is from the tail towards the head. Also in "Cosmic Superimposition", the flow of energy during sexual excitation is given as being upwards along the dorsal side, and down the ventral side from head towards the tail.

The Chinese physicians did not abstract the flow of energy, as Reich did. Their descriptions are in terms of the energy flow throughout the human body; the daily circulation of Ch'i. The time when each of the twelve organs comes to a maximum level of Ch'i was given as:

Lungs (03.0-05.0 a.m.)	Bladder (15.0-17.0 p.m.)
Large Intestine (05.0-07.0 a.m.)	Kidneys (17.0-19.0 p.m.)
Stomach (07.0-09.0 a.m.)	Heart Constrictor (19.0-21.0 p.m.)
Spleen-Pancreas (09.0-11.0 a.m.)	Three Heaters (21.0-23.0 p.m.)
Heart (11.0 a.m.-13.0 p.m.)	Gall Bladder (23.0 p.m.-01.0 a.m.)
Small Intestine (13.0-15.0 p.m.)	Liver (01.0-03.0 a.m.)

So we see that the idea of each organ pulsating in energy was described. Here, too, Reich was always stressing the application of the orgasm formula to the organ systems as well as to the total body.

The direction of the energy flow, as described by the Chinese, appears to go in the opposite direction from that described by Reich. According to Acupuncture, the main avenue of energy is from the pubic area to the chin, via the conception meridian (a main Yin sedation meridian), then from the mouth down to the anus via an internal pathway, then ascending to the head via the governor meridian (a main Yang stimulation meridian), to descend once more via a further internal pathway to the perineal area. Here is apparent disagreement, which needs to be explained.

45.   Reich, Wilhelm *Character Analysis* Moonday Press, U.S.A.

This separation leads to the Koch postulates of disease, which, until just the past few years, were accepted completely. The cause of disease is always sought in the exterior world, and not inside the body itself. An external agent is always thought to be the cause. This is in line with mechanistic reductionist science.

But recent developments have pointed away from this doctrine. The "Viral Oncogene" theory of Huebner and Todaro[46], and the "Provirus" theory of Temin[47], both assume that tumour viruses originate from normal cell constituents, under the influence of stress. Since these theories are important in guiding current cancer research, we must assume that a trend is being set.

On the other hand, both Acupuncture and Reich stress the internal factors in disease. To them, disease is primarily a situation body energy disequilibrium, and the most important factor in the treatment of disease is *diagnosis of the imbalance,* and steps leading to the return of normal energy conditions, homoeostasis.

Neither the Acupuncturists nor Reich treat the body as a collection of bits and pieces, but as a complete organism, which is a part of nature, in tune with the cosmos.

The consequence of the differing approach is not academic. One only has to compare the conventional cancer treatment, with its very elaborate equipment such as radiation therapy, to the orgone accumulator used by the Reichians, or the elaborate anaesthesia equipment, to the simple steel needle used for the same purpose by the Acupuncturist.

Both Acupuncture and Reich assume that the life energy enters the body from the outside; via food, solar energy, oxygen. This assumption is seen to flow from simple logic, since the energy necessary for life has to come from somewhere. Acupuncture says that the energy, Ch'i, is the mover, and mass follows as a result, as, for example in the circulation of the blood. Reich stressed the fact that the energy movements in the body are primary, and the

46.   Todaro, G. and Huebner, R. *The Viral Oncogene Hypothesis - New Evidence.*
        Proc. Nat. Acad. Sci. (U.S.A.) 69 1009 (1972)
47.   Temin, H.M. *The R.N.A. Tumor Viruses, Background and Foreground.*
        Proc. Nat. Acad. Sci. (U.S.A.) 69 1016 (1972)

biochemical changes are secondary, as, for example, the biochemical changes in schizophrenia.

The Chinese and Reich agree that the body energy flows. How the ancient Chinese reached this conclusion is unknown, but it seems that the physicians in antiquity reflected upon the state of energy in their own bodies.

It it not known when Acupuncture originated, but there are legends dating back to about 4,000 B.C., and certainly Acupuncture was practised in the Neolithic Age, using flints to apply pressure. We can, therefore, assume that the practice of Acupuncture dated back to the beginning of Chinese Civilization.

Tradition has it that the practice of Acupuncture began as the result of some accidental injury, which relieved pain in some other part of the body. But, in view of the dates, and the rich philosophical background, we would rather think of Acupuncture as being the result of an originally holistic way of thinking, a thought-process which considers the totality before looking at the specialities.

The Chinese system assumes two circulations of energy. The first is the superficial circulation of energy, Ch'i, through channels or *meridians,* and the second is a deep flow of energy.

The Chinese attribute disease to a disturbance in the functioning of the Ch'i. Since there is a flow of energy through each organ, the disturbed state of each organ is said to be due to either an excess of energy (too much Yang) or a deficiency of energy (too much Yin). Then the task of therapy becomes the restoration of proper energy functioning. The traditional doctor would use a variety of means such as Acupuncture, Tai Chi exercises, and herbal medication.

Reich described disease in similar terms. The pattern of disease was divided into two parts. One was due to a disturbance in the energy functioning of the body, called the *biopathies,* and the other class was one in which the disturbance to body energy came as a secondary result.

In the first category, such illnesses as cancer, cardiovascular troubles, hypertension, and asthma, would be included, and, in the second category, such things as the breaking of a bone due to mechanical injury, or infection from a communicable microbe. The two concepts of disease agree.

However, there is an fundamental tenet of Reich's concept, which is not extensively mentioned in Chinese works, the importance of sexuality. In Reich's concept, sexual repression is the central feature of biopathies. The Chinese did give great importance to the role of emotions in disease, but sexuality seems to have had a minor role.

To influence the flow of energy in the body, Acupuncture uses metal needles. There is frequently no known anatomical connection between the site of the needle and the organ to be affected. From the viewpoint of mechanistic biology, the situation is mysterious. We will attempt to answer in terms of the discoveries of Reich.

Reich discovered that a simple arrangement of metal and organic material in a box can lead to an environment in which the organism can obtain energy from the atmosphere. We will not go into the theory of how the accumulator works, except to say that the metal is assumed to attract and quickly repel the energy, in order to influence the direction and quantity of energy flow, so that a metal probe inserted in the body could influence the orgone concentrations.

In parallel, the Chinese believe that the function of the needle is to establish harmonious flow.

Of course, the language is different, but the basic idea in both approaches is to get pulsation going again in the organ, and dissipate the obstacles to these flows, the energy blocks.

We can assume that the energy blocks are tissues, where the energy itself is relatively immobile, or stale. Towards the end of his life, Reich worked out how stale energy could be influenced by simple configurations of metals and water, which could draw the energy away from such stagnant areas.

We are now in a position to attempt to understand the acupuncture techniques, in terms of the properties of the orgone energy. The needle can function to divert energy streams in the body, since the metal needles can influence the energy flow. We may also conceive of the metal needles being points, where the energy of the body is discharged. In this way, the needles would function to release metabolized orgone energy, which is not discharged in the normal way.

94

In this connection, it would be interesting to know if Acupuncture could be used for the so-called psychological troubles. There are now acupuncture treatments for various sexual malfunctions, such as erective impotence, and frigidity. Since these are commonly functions of character structure, it seems likely that Acupuncture could also be of more general value in psychiatry. In the treatment of drug addiction, needles can be used to relieve the withdrawal symptoms.

In the field of cancer, Acupuncture so far has been ineffective to our knowledge, except to relieve symptoms. From the view point of Reich, this inability may be understood.

According to his observations, Reich came to the conclusion that the basic cause of cancer was the contraction of the body energy field, the *shrinking biopathy*. He viewed cancer as a disease of the total body, with the affected organ merely being the weakest link in the chain.

The needles appear to cause a redistribution of the total body energy. If the overall energy level of the body is already too low, then the redistribution would not be of much help.

Reich observed that the impaired energy of the tissues was the result of a *long term chronic impaired breathing*. Since oxygen is the carrier of orgone in the atmosphere, the lowered oxygen supply would cause an energy deficiency.

Thinking in terms of Reich, Acupuncture could be of help in cancer prevention. If the needles were used to improve breathing, then the body would receive a greater oxygen supply, according to Reich[48], the disintegration process of the tissues would be retarded.

We have already mentioned that Reich discovered how to disperse configurations of stale energy. The techniques of DOR busting is extremely simple, and may be quickly demonstrated by holding a metal knife under running water, putting the point close to, but not touching, the area between the eyebrows.

After a few minutes, there will be a tugging sensation. Thus the energy field, being tugged, is the energy flow caused by the metal under running water. What we have constructed is a simple version of the DOR buster.

---

48.   Reich, Wilhelm *The Cancer Biopathy*. Moonday Press, U.S.A.

The application of this DOR buster technique, applied to acupuncture points, may attract cosmic energy to the organism via the acupuncture points, and thence for distribution throughout the whole system.

The orgone techniques offer ways of *getting energy into the body* by simple means, which do not require insertion of needles, whereas Acupuncture manipulates and regulates this energy. The combination of the two therapies could possibly produce the most powerful therapeutic weapon yet developed by man.

(This chapter was from an article written in conjunction with Professor Adolph Smith, Associate Professor of Physics, Sir George William University, Montreal.)

13　Electro-Acupuncture

I die by the help of too many physicians — ALEXANDER THE GREAT

IT WAS ONLY THIRTY YEARS AGO that Dr. Niboyet in France developed an instrument for measuring the variations of potential on the skin surface over the acupoints. Since that time, great strides have been made in the development of these instruments, and the interpretation of the many readings which can be taken with electro-energy acupuncture apparatus. Further research is being carried on in Russia, China, Japan, France, Germany and Roumania and other countries.

It has long been considered by the Chinese acupuncture experts that a large part of any failure in acupuncture therapy has been due to the fact that the needle has not been inserted in the correct position. The success of Acupuncture depends upon the insertion of the needle in the *exact* location of the correct point. It is not sufficient to make a correct assessment of Yin and Yang, and an exact diagnosis, and the perfect selection of the acupoint. All this is of no avail, unless the point is stitched at the exact spot.

The two most difficult arts to master in the learning of Acupuncture are pulse diagnosis and point location. Even the experienced Chinese physician, who has studied and practised for many years, uses some degree of personal and subjective interpretation. Locating points precisely is difficult, and is a technique which cannot easily be acquired by western practitioners, who are accustomed to a quick scientific approach, easy diagnosis and therapy.

It was from this need that electro-acupuncture developed, and, using it, physicians are not only able to locate the acupoint accurately, but are also able to make other assessments, which the Chinese, with their traditional methods, have been unable to do.

The discharge of a condensor over acupoints is considerably steeper than that over the neutral skin, and, from this, it was deduced that the Chinese points were, in fact, pores of an electro-magnetic character in the skin.

Electro-acupuncture provides the following opportunities:

a) To establish overall basic values for the vital-energy flow in the body. (Traditional Acupuncture assesses these subjectively.)

b) The diversities of the left and right side of the body can be measured and assessed. (This, too, traditional Acupuncture does only subjectively.)

c) It allows measurements of the vital-energy flow at different points of the meridian, and, therefore, shows just where the Yin and Yang equilibrium breaks down. (Traditional Chinese medicine cannot do this.)

d) It gives an indication of the degree of organic disease in the meridians, which can be read off the metre.

e) It is able to give indication that an organ's function is impaired, and will, if not treated, develop into organic disease.

f) It has also a therapeutic application.

g) By being able to record readings, treatment by treatment, objective proof of Yin-Yang balance alteration may be obtained.

h) It gives an exact location of the acupoints.

i) Finally, it opens up a vast area of scientific procedure, to make Acupuncture less subjective, and a more objectively-demonstrable practice.

The apparatus used indicates the location of the acupoints, by means of a magic eye. This shutter is built into a hand electrode held by the practitioner, who locates the acupoints by brushing the instrument lightly over the surface of the skin near the location of the point. The patient holds the neutral electrode in his hand. On approaching the point, the shutter should close. The sensitivity of the shutter is regulated by means of a knob, which has a scale reading. If set too high, then the magic shutter will operate over the whole of the skin area, and, if it is set too low, then it will not operate at all. It is, therefore, necessary to set the machine at the patient's own mean sensitivity.

If the shutter comes sharply to a close, it indicates that the probe is over an acupoint. By exerting pressure with the probe, a slight indentation is made on the skin. This mark gives an exact location for needle stitching. Voltage, current and frequency at which the instrument works are such that no injuries can come to the patient.

Diagnosis, using electro-acupuncture, enables a practitioner to measure the energy value of the acupoints, and this method is so subtle that incipient changes in the energy patterns of organs can be assessed, so that an early diagnosis can be made at a time when the patient is as yet unaware of any trouble. This early diagnosis makes it easier for the practitioner to use preventive medicine in his practice.

With the apparatus, the currents sent into the body meet, in reaction, the bio-electric currents which each organ generates. To understand this, one has only to think of the E.C.G. and the E.E.G. The result of the encounter of the patient's bio-electric force, and the current of the machine, gives the measured value.

From this, it can be appreciated that the machine will locate the acupoints precisely, because the latter express a reduced cutaneous and subcutaneous resistance in relation to the surrounding tissue.

Modern electro-acupuncture practice has built up a clinical differential diagnosis from assessing the reducing variant drops on the indicator of the acupoint machine. The valuation of the variants is supplied by our knowledge of the abnormal physiological inter-connections of the individual ailments.

Another interesting procedure which can be performed with electro-acupuncture apparatus is the diagnosis of potential disease on each side of the body. With the twelve paired meridians, it can be assessed quickly whether the disease is in the right or left organ, or on the right or left side of a single organ.

For example, if, on taking readings on the lung meridian, it is found that the right-sided reading shows a slow climb, then it can be deduced that there is functional impairment on the right lung. Also, if, on the next reading on the left meridian, there is a maximum reading and a fast drop, it can be deduced that the left lung is organically diseased, the extent of which would be recognizable by the speed of the decline. In this way, functional or organic impairment can be distinguished.

When investigating single organs, such as the liver or the stomach, the method indicates malfunction of different sections of the organ. In the stomach area, for example, we can learn of the condition of the fundus and the small curvature, as against the pyloris. In the large intestine, we can distinguish between various conditions of the ascending or descending areas. In the case of appendicitis, there is a fall of the meter of the electro-acupuncture apparatus, when one probe is placed on the right side of the small intestine meridian.

If the indicator on the machine climbs very slowly during investigations, it is a sign of functional disturbance. The organ is shown to be "tired", and is using much needed reserves to match electrically the test current.

When there is organic damage, the indicator rises and then drops. This shows that the current cannot be met and held. According to the speed of the fall, we can assess the extent of the organic damage.

With the instrument, it is possible to test the value of each single acupoint in the course of the meridian, in order to make a survey of the vital energy flow in the meridian. By this method, it is possible to assess at which point on the meridian any block in its flow might occur. The method used is as follows: – the terminal reading of the meridian is taken, plus one or two other readings along the meridian. If these readings are equal, then it may be assumed that the energy flows through the meridian are unimpaired. If, however, there are different readings, then the point of the blockage can be traced.

By taking the gross readings on the left and right side of bilateral meridians, the state of the vital activity on the two different circuits of each bilateral meridian can be assessed. The readings on the suspect circuits can be compared with the readings on the more healthy circuits, and a quantitative evaluation of hyper- and hypo-Yang or Yin activity can be made. This provides an objective indication for the use of the needles.

14   The Kirlian Effect

Man is Heaven and Earth in miniature – CHINESE PROVERB

KIRLIAN WAS BORN AND WORKED in the U.S.S.R. In 1939, he discovered the effect or aura, now known as *Kirlian*. Scientists in the U.S.S.R. are striving to produce more and more evidence to prove the validity of this phenomenon. The method is described by the Russians as a process which converts non-electrical properties of an object or area into electrical effects, which can then be filmed, by means of high voltage spark discharges.

Laszlo[49] claims that Kirlian photography and Acupuncture will eventually take their place amongst the new sciences called "Systems Research". This is a form of development from the life sciences, such as behaviour, biology, bio-physics, sociology, physiology, etc. *Systems Research* is a new science, which combines under the one heading all the life sciences, just as *physics* is an umbrella term for all non-life sciences.

Fuller[50], explains and describes the behavioural relationships, and mutual co-operative interactions, of living organisms, acting for their common good, and, in such a way as to be over and above the integrity of any one of its component parts.

This, of course, happens also in the non-organic world. There is still no explanation of how chemical compounds organize themselves into molecules, or how they hold together in groups, in consistent prescribed relationships, any more than there is any explanation of how biological cells come together to form animal or plant tissue.

The Kirlian aura demonstrates that all matter has a 'flare' pattern. Organic matter has a *changing* flare pattern, whereas non-organic matter has a constant pattern. With organic matter, the flare of any one animal or plant cannot be explained by the form or the flare of any of its parts. The flare of the whole is exclusive to the whole, and exclusive to that particular moment.

49.   Laszlo, E. *Introduction to Systems Philosophy*. New York, Gordon and Breach 1972.
50.   Fuller, R.B. *Intuition*. New York. Doubleday and Co., 1972.

Neither can the flare of the subject under investigation be likened to the flare pattern of the species of the subject; each aura is unique to the subject, and unique to that moment.

If we are to adopt Fuller's term 'synergy', then the Kirlian effect is visual proof of such an effect. In the same way, when we take the acupuncture pulses, those pulses are unique, at that instant, only to that patient alone. This fact is of great importance to the Acupuncturist, because it tells us why pulses vary from moment to moment.

If the treatment is successful, the synergetic effect will vary, and the pulses will vary during the treatment. The principle behind the synergetic effect utterly belies the idea that Acupuncture is nerve impulse control. Slowly, but certainly, the new sciences take us back, deeper and deeper, into acupuncture history and philosophy.

Another most important discovery shown by Kirlian photography is the 'phantom leaf' effect[51]. In this, a part of a leaf has been cut out, and the leaf is repeatedly photographed, for example every five minutes. The whole leaf is still visible in the photograph for some time afterwards. But, as the rest of the leaf dies, the phantom effect diminishes and, finally, disappears.

We, as Acupuncturists, recognize this phantom effect, on patients who have lost an organ, for we can still read the "phantom" pulse.

For years, this has been ridiculed, for how can you read a pulse relating to something in the body, which is no longer visible? This point of view has been put forward by the antagonists, as evidence that acupuncture pulses are nonsense. We have known the effect, and have insisted that the pulse does exist. Now, with Kirlian photography and the idea of the synergetic effect, we have visible evidence that it is feasible, and, indeed, probable, that the pulse can and does exist when a body organ is lost. The overall synergetic effect remains, with or without the organ, so long as the subject remains alive, just as with the phantom leaf effect. (The photographed leaf, of course, has already been detached from the tree, so that it would die in any case.)

In the Kirlian photograph, for example, from a finger tip[52], there is a great difference between the photographs when the subject is calm as against

51.   Moss, T. and Johnson K. *Radiation Field Photography.* Psychic 1972. Pages 50-54.
52.   Moss, T. *Searching for Psi* Psychic 1971 - 2. Pages 40-44.

when he is tense; the more the tension, the more the flare intensifies and changes colour. Healers have been known to give off great auras of a bluish tint. It is interesting how the colour blue keeps recurring throughout so many reports concerning these new sciences. People who have claimed to see auras, have always maintained that healthy subjects give off a bluish aura. The more ill a subject is, the more grey it becomes. Kirlian pictures verify these statements. We can now produce visual evidence to substantiate what the aura-seeing people have stated for a hundred years. Many researchers believe that the Kirlian effect is a method of photographing bio-energy, defined by the Czechoslovakian parapsychologists as a form of energy-force, which is more subtle than electro-magnetic waves. It is associated with the living organism, in the form of psychic waves, impulses and components, such as in E.S.P., bird migration, intuition, and the other forms of cosmic communication used by all animals, under the most diverse conditions.

Von Bertanlaffy, in his General Systems Theory, postulates that all organisms fall into a special category, which he terms "an open-ended system". Open-ended systems keep up a constant exchange with the environment. An open-ended system, a living organism, is constantly replacing worn-out material, maintaining a state of equilibrium both inside and outside its own physical circumference—a ceaseless flow of information to and from the environmental cosmos. The system is not passive, but always, intrinsically, active.

Krippner[53] likened this to a gyroscope, saying "the well functioning, fully developed person is a human gyroscope, who maintains both an internal and external balance with a series of forces and energies".

The position taken up by these various scientists is very similar to the position that I have been taking up in these lectures, and it is exciting to find that researchers are coming to similar conclusions, although each approaches the subject from his own angle.

It is not my intention in this talk to go into the details of what constitutes Kirlian photographic apparatus, or explain how the system works, as there is ample literature available on how to make one, and exactly how it works, as far as it is understood. Sufficient to say that it is a high voltage

53.   Krippner, S. and Rubin, D. *The Kirlian Aura*. Anchor Books, New York 1974.

alternating current field of energy-like waves, caught between two condensor plates, which takes an aura-type picture of anything which appears between the plates, when the curren is used — a type of electrical photograph. The term adopted by many of the Soviet scientists, to describe the Kirlian effect as 'bio-plasma'. Others claim that it is a cold-electron discharge which is photographed, and not a human aura at all.

I am not prepared, nor do I have the knowledge, to enter into the dispute. The physicists, who are concerned with Acupuncture, with E.S.P., what we term the *pro-life scientists,* accept willingly the synergetic concept, and the fact that auras are being photographed. I can only add that the photographs do change with changing moods; certain colours do appear; the discharge does diminish during illness, and changes drastically after death. The phantom effect does exist; there is a unique discharge over the Acupuncture points, which is constant in position, but is ever-changing in colour and intensity.

Whatever the final decision of just what constitutes the Kirlian effect, one thing appears certain, that it must enhance the case for Acupuncture, as Acupuncture is involved with the overall synergy in nature.

Moss says that bio-plasma is similar, if not identical, to the aura of the astral body, spoken of in yogic teaching. This was also put forward by Inyushin[54] who suggested that the negatively-charged electrons react to a changing magnetic field.

But Adamenko[55] said that they are cold electron emissions, which can give us important information concerning the very nature of organic materials. The cold electron theorists suggest that the field around all matter, which is photographed, represents electrons, which are away from the surface, with ever-differing velocity. They say that it is this discharge which is photographed, which they call the cold electron emission.

Pressman[56], also a Russian, postulated that whole organisms are more sensitive to electro-magnetic fields than the individual parts of the organism. Further, he suggested that this sensitivity is an organizational sensitivity, and

54.   Inyushin, V.M. *On the Biological Essence of the Kirlian Effect.*
      Alma-Ata, Kazakj, U.S.S.R. Kazakj University 1968.
55.   Adamenko, V.G. *Electrodynamics of Living Systems.* Journal of Paraphysics,
      Volume 4, No. 4. 1970. Downtown, Wiltshire, England. Pages 113-120.
56.   Pressman, A.S. *The Role of Electromagnetic Fields in Vital Processes.* Biofizika 1964. Gilz.

essential to life. Pressman is convinced that the understanding of these electro-magnetic fields will depend upon a social investigation of communities rather than the investigation of single organisms.

We are aware that the modern tendency in science is to attempt to understand a system by examining isolated parts of that system. But this ignores the wholeness of the organism's structure, and the essential relationship of the parts to the whole, the whole to the parts, the parts to the parts, and the whole to the cosmos. The approach is a largely self-defeating exercise, for, while it continues to prove bits and pieces, inevitably it misses what life is about.

Lakatos [57] said "For centuries, knowledge has meant proven knowledge, proven either by the power of the intellect, or by the evidence of the senses. The terms of proof were questioned by sceptics two thousands years ago, but this challenge was beaten into confusion by the glory of Newtonian physics. Einstein's work again turned the tables, and now very few philosophers or scientists still think that scientific knowledge is, or can be, proven knowledge. Few people realize that, with this development, the whole classical structure of intellectual values falls in ruins, and has to be replaced".

Returning to the discussion of what happens with a Kirlian photograph 'phantom leaf' effect, when the photograph reveals a picture of the whole leaf some considerable time after a piece of the leaf has been severed, Adamenko is of the opinion that the traditional channels in the leaf are so numerous that there is an enormous redundancy of information, so much so that the essential structure of the leaf remains, even beyond the time when a portion has been removed. A similar situation arises when a finger-print is removed from a subject's skin. The Kirlian photograph still shows the original finger-print.

Inyushin, who developed the idea of the bioplasma, suggests that there is a single integrated system of elementary charge particles, which are always dominant, as long as the organism is alive. This will produce a constant minimum pattern or aura, even after a limb has been severed, a finger-print has been sanded away, or a part of a leaf has been cut away. He claims that this is different from the emission of inorganic material, which does not change, and must be distinguished as being different.

57. Lakatos, I., Meeting of the Aristotelian Society. London, England. October 1968.

It is organizational, non-chaotic, and integrated. Its entropy is almost non-existent. In other words, one can almost say that the bioplasma in the living organism *cares,* whereas the emission from inorganic material has no integrated structural integrity, and it exists because it exists, there being no heirarchy, and no attempt to cohere from an organizational standpoint. If a cut takes place, this the photograph will show.

Tiller[58] makes some excellent points, when summarizing his view on energy fields. He says that man can anticipate extending his horizons into new domains of awareness and perception regarding nature. These new concepts need not, in any way, deny many of the old concepts of man, or of the universe, nor need they be a threat to conventional physics. Professor Tiller's views do not agree, however, with many leading scientists.

Newton was, in no way, shown to be wrong by the discoveries of Einstein, but his ideas were shown to be *limited* to particular aspects of gravitation. Tiller, discussing work carried out in the U.S.S.R., suggests some interesting points, and he says that psychokineses, healers, and acupuncture practitioners are dealing with energy fields completely different from the ones recognized by particle physics.

Experiments, he says, show us that there is a level of energy which is magnetic, as distinct from electrical; that there is, in organic material, an organizing rather than a disorganizing tendency, for example temperature *increases,* thereby seemingly violating the second law of thermodynamics. There is a radiational pattern of energy, an aura, which is a force-envelope around organic substance, which relate to the organism wholeness.

There is growing evidence from a multitude of experiments with plants, animals and humans, that there is intercommunication, which is continuous, at various levels, between all things in the universe. There is evidence that there exist energy manifestations at different levels which are unique to each energy pattern, and stable at each level, in uncharted time-space relationships, with more and more evidence pointing to the idea that there are time and space waves unique to the minds, the life-force, and the life-energy. In fact, with understanding of these unique time-space relationships, which tie all minds into the cosmic whole, it but remains to tune in to the universal consciousness.

58.   Tiller, Professor W. *The Kirlian Aura.* Stamford University, U.S.A. 1973.

15 Magnets

What is the most difficult of all? What seems the easiest to you: to see with your eyes what lies before your eyes — GOETHE

OVER THE LAST FEW YEARS, it has become more and more real to me that Acupuncture must work by way of electro-magnetic and gravitational forces. My own feeling, supported by the results of many researchers, has ever-increasingly pointed in this direction — dowsing, homoeopathy, the vital force in nature-cure, E.S.P., bio-energetics, Uri Geller's apparent powers, astrology, herbal medicine, Schussler salts, psychic healers, macrobiotics, Bach remedies, Bio-salts, radionics, auras, Kirlian photography, the teachings of Krishnamurti, Psychosynthesis, Zen, Gestalt, Encounter, the research of Reich, Eeman, Lakhovsky, the laying on of hands, bird migration, the trans-ocean movement of fish, bio-rhythms, colour therapy, radiesthesia, and many others.

All these researches, diagnostic aids, and therapies, could not all be wrong; we cannot all be deluding ourselves, and all the patients getting well cannot *all* have been only psychosomatic cases, particularly when small children and animals have been helped. So many orthodox diagnoses, subsequently denied, could not all have been wrong in the first place.

Why has there been so much opposition to these non-material ideas? It could not be because they were unorthodox, because many of these systems of healing were developed by orthodox medical men. I believe that the opposition stemmed from the concept that, to accept the validity of these therapies would throw into doubt much of the scientific thought of the day.

To accept the principles behind these concepts would mean breaking away from the traditional chemical premise, and would revolutionize the whole of modern medical concepts. It would mean admitting, once and for all, that there is more to life than chemicals.

It would mean admitting that modern instruments could never tell us what life is, which might bring about a loss of face for some very learned authorities. As long as scientists can continue to examine material substances, they can know when they are on the right road. They believe that, with enough research, they will be able to know it all.

But these new approaches belie this belief, and the dedicated researchers suspect that one admission would bring a flood of new ideas, which could sweep away all the cherished tradition, and, possibly, invalidate all the training. For, if something is not chemical, and cannot be traced by chemical means, or by electronic means, how can it be measured or examined?

For the traditional scientist, with his long history of material research, the impossibility of proof seems too great a pill to swallow. For the moment, it is more comfortable to remain unconvinced. In recent years, there has been an ever-increasing quantity of evidence relating to various unorthodox therapies, and the strange phenomena which take place in the cosmos, in the world, with plants, animals and man. How can we talk to plants? How can we know what someone a thousand miles away is thinking? How can Uri Geller bend metal? How can untrained people in the Phillipines perform successful operations without knives, or with rusty ones? These unanswerables abound, and there comes a time when even the most materially-based people must wonder, and many scientists have begun to question further.

Modern medicine owes much of its present dilemma to the upsurge of publicity about Acupuncture. The Chinese used Acupuncture successfully for anaesthesia, and this could not be either explained or ignored.

Most medical men are dedicated, honest practitioners. But it *is* hard, after years of study, and often many years in practice, being highly respected in society, perhaps achieving great eminence, to be told that their whole approach is limited in application. For hundreds of years, orthodox medicine has held absolute power. They have been researching, and teaching, according to their highest ideals. Let us be grateful that medical men are honest, and have their patients' needs foremost in their minds, even above their own comfort and well-being, and that, therefore, they will be willing to change their view, if what we say is proved to their satisfaction to be correct.

From the established medical world's standpoint, we are upstarts with little money, no standing, no recognized training, no government backing, no orthodox medical background, yet we say *Stop, you are wrong, listen to us.*

108

When the first orthodox doctors became interested in Acupuncture, it was not surprising that they set out to prove that Acupuncture was a combination of nerve impulses and chemical reactions, and that, therefore, it could be fitted into orthodox theory. But, from my viewpoint, I cannot accept this.

We look to traditional Chinese ideas, look to all the natural therapies, the unexplainable phenomena around us, and recognize that there must be more to life than chemistry.

Can we, in one concept, bind all these unorthodox approaches together? If once we can do that, we will be performing a great service to mankind, and also a service to all practitioners and followers of non-orthodox medicine.

It is my belief that there is an underlying principle, which binds them all together, and that this principle is electro-magnetism, one of the *bridging* mechanisms, standing between pure energy and chemistry. If we begin to think and work along these lines, many 'insolubles' begin to fall into place.

Postulating that the body is an open-ended circuit, as far as electro-magnetic forces are concerned, the use of magnetism should have an effect which can be measured, and we should be able to influence the state of health, by the use of magnets.

With this in mind, a few years ago, I used my first magnet on a patient, a 300-guass flat ferrite magnet, measuring an inch and a quarter by three eighths by a quarter of an inch.

The patient had been treated for trigeminal neuralgia, which had been intractable over eight years. He was mathematics professor at a Canadian University, and had undergone numerous forms of treatment, to no effect. We, ourselves, treated him six or eight times, again to no effect, using osteopathy, traditional acupuncture, and diet. It was then that I used my first magnet, strapped to his face with a piece of elastoplast. In twenty minutes, the pain was gone, never to return, we hope.

I thought that I had discovered something new, but there is nothing new. I found out that there have been conventions for magnet healing in the United States since 1960[59], I also discovered that two books had been

---

59.   Davis, R.A. and Rawls, W.C. *Magnetism and its Effect on the Living System.*
      Exposition Press, Hicksville, New York 1974.

published in India[60], also a series of works in Japan[61], and that there was a compulsive magnet worker and healer, also in the United States. I was not alone, nor had I discovered anything new, but it was a revelation and a new avenue opening to me.

From my very limited experience, I have subsequently made a few deductions. I consider that acupuncture treatment must influence the electro-magnetic forces in the body, and magnetic stimulation helps to rectify body imbalance. By re-zoning healthy magnetic vibrations through the organism, I believe that the energy of the body tunes into these vibrations, and vibrates out the unwanted oscillations, which permits the chemical repair of the body.

In my opinion, magnet healing is divided into two basic forms, excluding Acupuncture. The first is the actual use of magnets, and the second the laying on of hands, the strange power which Hippocrates referred to, *and his patients got better.*

Ewart[62] reported that micro-organisms such as ciliate flagellate had been placed in a strong magnetic field; when the field was in line with the movement of the microbes, nothing was noted; but when the field was placed at right angles to the movement of the microbes, their velocity slowed down.

Jennison[63] reported that certain yeast fungi had their bud formation reduced as much as thirty percent when placed in a 3,000 gauss magnetic field. Nakagawa[64] cultured B coli within, and outside, a magnetic field. The B coli in the magnetic field were noticeably more prolific within twenty-four hours. A Dr. Hayashi subsequently repeated this experiment, with similar results; but, additionally, he discovered that, if the direction of movement of the bacilli was perpendicular to that of the magnetic field, their movement

60. Davis and Bhattacharya *Magnet and Magnetic Fields.* Mukhopodhyay, Calcutta 1970.
61. Fuzimoto, S. *The Magnetic Band.* "Aimante." Internal Dept. Red Cross Hospital, Kyoto, Japan 1963.
   Nakagawa and others. *Biological Effects of Magnetic Fields.* Dept. of Int. Med., Isuza Hospital, Tokyo, Japan 1963.
62. Ewart, A.J. *On the Physics and Physiology of Protoplasmic Streaming in Plants.* Clarendon Press 1903.
63. Jennison, M.W. *Journal of Bacteriology.* 1937 Volume 33. Pages 15-16
64. Nakagawa *Journal of Japanese Society of Internal Medicine.* 1958. Volume 47-1, Page 74.

was more restricted than those which were cultured outside the magnetic field. Sswastin[65] noted a similar phenomenon with algae. When the field was positioned perpendicular to their streaming, the protoplasm even became extinct. He also proved that wheat could be made to bud much faster by using magnetic forces.

A great deal of research has been carried out on the influence of magnetic fields. In fact, over four hundred papers on the subject have been delivered and published during the last hundred years.

Many varied effects have been recorded relating to plants and animals. Lenzi[66] reported that there was no change produced in surface tension in blood serum in an electric field, but that the blood sedimentation rate was increased. With very strong magnetism, giant cells may be produced, and chromosomes connected to each other have resulted in a symmetric nitosis.

Many conflicting conclusions have been reached in relation to magnetic fields. Some scientists say nitosis is affected; blood cells are affected adversely; or beneficially; or, even, not at all.

Up to the tenth century, magnetism was widely used in medicine. It then appeared to have been forgotten.

With the return of interest in this century, until about 1960, medical reports were critical, and its efficacy was considered nil, even adverse. But, recently, experiments with the use of magnets appear to be more favourably reported.

Hansen[67] in Sweden successfully used magnets for the treatment of lumbago, sciatica, and arthritis, without pathological changes. The south pole of the magnet was used over the affected part for ten to forty minutes a day for twelve days. No magnetic strength was recorded for these experiments.

During this century, there have been various attempts to evaluate magnetism for plant growth and for healing. The 1970's are seeing magnet healing introduced into Acupuncture, which is its rightful place.

65. Sswastin, P.W. *Planta* 11. Pages 683-720. 1930.
66. Lenzi, M. *Strahlentherapie*. 1940. 67. Pages 219-250.
67. Hansen, K.M. *Acta Medica Scandinavica*. 1938. 97. Pages 339-364.

Dr. Bhattarcharya has said "Man is composed of billions of cells, each of which is an electrical unit in itself. These cells are vibrating at specific frequencies. The cells pick up their vibrations from the atmosphere, the source of all frequencies. The earth is a huge magnet, and it is radiating magnetic energy to all things, human, animal, plant, etc. From this concept, it can be assumed that the magnet must have a special benefit for every living thing". I like this statement, and how well it fits in with acupuncture philosophy.

My own thinking about the use of magnets moved towards my eastern philosophic approach. It seemed that many researchers were already using the magnet in this way, but, from experience, and not from a philosophical concept. It appeared that I had an immediate advantage, and so it proved to be.

After considering the subject in relation to the overall yin and yang picture, I began to use the magnets over the centre of the area of pain or illness, using the south pole of the magnet when I wanted to stimulate, and the north pole when sedation was required. In one or two cases, I made mistakes, and the patient was made temporarily worse by the treatment. In one particular case, I relaxed an osteo-arthritic hip, using the magnet north pole point over the affected area, ignoring, at the same time, that the patient was in a state of deep depression, which was exacerbated. It was some three weeks before this unfortunate *side-effect* abated. This reminded me forcefully that I must never get carried away, and fail to consider the *whole* condition, such a very basic tenet of acupuncture.

But so many other results were most encouraging. A patient in the clinic at Tyringham arrived on a Saturday with migraine, which was treated by cold compresses, massage to the cervicals, osteopathy, acupuncture, relaxation, rest in a darkened room, even *migrail* was administered, but all to no avail. On the Tuesday at 5.00 p.m., the senior sister reported that the patient was beginning to vomit blood, and a haemhorrage looked possible. I was called, applied a magnet to the forehead. By 6.30 p.m., the patient awakened without migraine, hopefully never to return.

On some occasions, our initial use of the magnet had no effect; but improvement took place after changing the polarity.

A patient with chronic osteo-arthritis of both knees, which was very resistant to treatment, made a recovery after using ring magnets over the knees. We have since treated about two hundred cases with magnets, and have seen satisfactory results in well over sixty-five percent of them. Gradually, we hope to extend our knowledge and our range.

Davis found that, in rats, cancer tumours reduced in size, or disappeared, when subjected to the north pole of the magnet. He explains another experiment whereby red blood-cells are magnetized, and can be observed spinning in a polarized circular direction. If the magnets are reversed, the spin direction reverses, which would seem to indicate there there is a directional flow emanating from the magnet.

A further experiment conducted by Davis conflicts with the orthodox view that the flow of the magnetic force moves from one pole to the other in a semi-circular movement. By taking a pin, and gently sliding it along the length of the magnet, in the centre, a spot will be reached where there is no magnetic pull. At this point, there is neutrality. If the force of the magnet is proportional to the electron charge and spin, then, at this point, where there is *no* magnetic charge, the spin must be at the point between reversing directions. This would explain the reversal of the movement of the red blood cells, when the poles of the magnet are reversed.

Davis claims that the vortex of the electrons, the spin, changes its direction by a one hundred and eighty degree turn, and then carries on in the same direction. When leaving the south pole of the magnet, which is the energizing side, the yang side, the vortex is spinning in a clockwise direction. After reaching the centre of power, it reverses by a hundred and eighty degrees, and carries on towards the north pole, in an anti-clockwise, the yin, direction, and this, in our terms, is the sedating side.

It became evident to me that the whole concept of electro-magnetism was tying in with my personal concepts of Acupuncture. Where the meridians change from yin to yang, and yang to yin, are they not doing exactly the same as the flat magnet? Could the meridians be forms of electro-magnet forces?

Let us examine what would happen if this were the case. The Heart meridian, yin, pairs up with the Small Intestine meridian, yang. Unlike poles attract, so that the magnetism from Heart 9 would be attracted to Small Intestine 1. The positive, yang, Small Intestine point would attract the magnetic form from the end point of the yin sedating meridian. From the yang Small Intestine, it would be attracted to the yin Bladder meridian, and so on, right through all the meridians, and eventually connect back to the Heart meridian, thus completing the entire body circuit.

How does the yang meridian get its "yangness"?

Yang, being positive, draws into itself the centrifugal force. The points of the yang meridians draw in energy from the cosmos, attracting the energy. This energy is charged with light at the points, as demonstrated by Kim Bong Han. A form of photo-synthesis takes place. The light, together with the cosmos energy, becomes vitalized in the body, becoming our vital energy, our life energy.

As already outlined in this series of lectures, the energy is metabolized in the organism. The sour Ch'i, the dead energy, is then discharged via the yin meridian points, on the yin meridians. It may be that light, in some way, allows the metabolized energy to be discharged.

According to this theory, the slightest disturbance at any point would cause a disarrangement in the vortex directional flow of the magnetic force in the meridian. The acupuncture needle could clear the spin disturbance, and set the magnetic charge oscillating in correct balance once again, turning into all the meridians.

This idea becomes clearer if it is remembered that the electro-magnetic gravitational charges involved are very small, 0.4 of a gauss being equal to the gravitational pull. The charge picked up by the needle from the cosmos may also be very small, possibly one hundredth of a gauss, perhaps even less.

We may, therefore, be thinking in terms of a homoeopathic electro-magnetic dose. May be one millionth of a gauss. This could well be enough force to change the vortex directional flow, thereby correcting the yin yang flow, which may be flowing incorrectly due to a meridian blockage, the needles attracting some energy from the cosmos, and sending it into the meridians.

The pulse and the symptomatic patient-picture feeds us with the necessary information as to which points may be in trouble.

The acupuncture pulses are a form of vibrational oscillation build-up from the magnetic electron movement, building up to firm inner vibration, like a body rhythmic mantra, a natural mantra; just as the noise heard in one's ears, when all is silent, is a body mantra; a coming-together of the body rhythms, building up into a form of echo.

I could go deeply into the use of magnets for the treatment of disease, and explain how it is being used successfully for almost every ailment, but I would rather spend our time discussing how we can utilize magnetism in our work as Acupuncturists.

My next step was to magnetize acupuncture needles, and use them therapeutically. This proved more difficult than expected, for it was almost impossible to find any needle which could be magnetized. In the end, I magnetized sewing needles. They were thick, and a little painful in use, but worked. The results were encouraging. But it was not possible to use these needles for many of the points, because of their thickness. My work was confined mainly to Colon 4, as it is such a useful and important point, and easily accessible. Besides using the magnetized needle on Colon 4, I used other needles at the same treatment, and I have no doubt in my own mind that the results were dramatically improved. Unfortunately, my needles rotted in spirit, and I knew that to continue would be dangerous, and I had to abandon my project.

Then I discovered a French needle which will take a low power of magnetism, about twelve gauss. I had these magnetized, and have been using them on selected patients with excellent success in each case.

A lady patient with chronic sinusitis had been treated by diet and conventional acupuncture with limited success. There was a great deal of pain, and the patient was very distressed. (I would point out here that it is very unusual not to have success in the treatment of sinusitis with acupuncture, but this case was the exception.) The patient returned in distress, and we decided to use the magnetized needles. The relief was immediate, the patient was able to breathe well, felt a clearness in the head, and said that she felt as if there had been a scraping of the sinuses. I could go on to discuss many more cases, but I trust that I have made my point.

My thinking is that the magnetic needle was used to magnetically cleanse the meridian, and balance vortex flow and rhythm. If a magnet is placed in a yin meridian, such as the heart, with its north pole into the acupuncture point, it will repel the magnetic force in the meridian, and this must move it along the meridian, thereby clearing it, breaking down blockages. It will further break down congestion, relax the meridian life-energy, producing a yin effect. If the south pole of the magnet is used, then, through the skin, it attracts energy from the cosmos, into the meridian, a yang effect.

The yang cosmic energy is powerful, and, even when the yang point of the needle is used on a yang meridian, it still produces a yang effect, by driving the cosmic energy into the repelling meridians.

The north end of the needle, yin, on a yang meridian, produces a yin effect, because the yang of the meridian, being stronger than the yin, will escape into the cosmos, with the needle thus *yinanizing* the meridian.

At first, I only used magnetized needles on selected acupuncture points, according to the normal laws, but I now also use the end points. My reasoning here is that, if I use a yin-magnetized needle at the end point of a yin meridian, not only will it force the charge along the meridian by repelling it, but it will also attract the force from the adjoining meridian, as yin will attract yang, negative attracts positive, and the north pole of the magnet attracts the south pole of the meridian. A great deal of further research and thinking needs to be done along these lines:

> as to the best gauss to have on the needle.
> as to the best length for needles for different meridians.
> Should the gauss be stronger on the more complicated meridians, such as the bladder meridian?
> Should the magnetism be pulsed in, or come from a static point?
> If it is going to be pulsed, what frequency, what gauss?
> How many gauss exist in a meridian?
> Should the charge vary from meridian to meridian?
> Does the meridian charge vary between health and disease? If so, can this be a new and important diagnostic procedure?
> Does the gauss change with the length of the needle?
> Does the charge vary during the day, with moon or climatic changes?
> Is the meridian gauss charge stable?

As the gausses are so small and they are neutralized and altered so easily, they must be constantly measured and adjusted. To answer most of these problems, a magnetometer is required.

I have tried to trace my thinking during the last few years, as I have become concerned that Acupuncture might become lost to orthodox thinking. It was not until I began to investigate magnetism, that I felt that I had some form of an answer. I trust that you will agree with me that we need never again be concerned with allowing anyone to repeat that Acupuncture is a chemical function. The cosmos is teeming with energy, an inexhaustible supply, which the techniques of Acupuncture can tap.

Nanbu[68], and a team of workers, treated 1,163 stiff-shouldered patients, who were each given a magnetic band to wear on the arm, 642 acting as controls. (The placebo patients had each been given a special magnetic band, so that, if they tested it with, for example, a pin, on the outside, it would lift the pin, but there was no magnetism on the inside, which came into contact with the patient.) The treatment was considered successful if the pain had *completely disappeared in one week* after the commencement of the treatment. The result was that 476 of the treated patients (40.9%) benefitted, compared with 41 (6.4%) of the placebo patients.

Interesting and illuminating though this report was, it seemed that the magnets in this experiment were being used in a haphazard manner. They were not related to the area of pain, nor were they used with any discernible standard, e.g. according to the north or south poles, the negative or positive, the yin or yang. This led me to look further.

The first reports I read concerning the use of magnets which really appealed to me as an Acupuncturist, came in two books already quoted from, by Dr. Bhattacharya, He says, further "The south pole, being hot in character, is energizing in nature, while the north pole, being cold in character, has a retarding effect". Perfect yin and yang. He says that true to Indian philosophy "The five elements are to be found in the poles of a magnet. These elements are earth, fire, water, air and ether. The north pole is constituted of the forces of earth and water, the south pole of fire and the neutral zone of air and ether". Again, this fits in with our concept. We only need to substitute 'wood' and 'metal' for 'air' and 'ether'.

68.   Nanbu, Japanese Tobata National Railway Hospital 1960.

Dr. Battacharya uses magnet dowsing to determine many subtle vibrations in the organism, including a kind of answering service of "yes" and "no", as one would call the spirits, using a yin and yang type of question; he uses magnets to determine a person's possible life-line; bio-energetic rhythm; colour therapy, jewel therapy, determining which jewel gives off beneficial radiations.

In addition, Dr. Battacharya uses magnet dowsing to determine disease indications in a subject; which homoeopathic remedies to use; which vitamins; the actual cause and seat of any disease; the likelihood of recovery; the patient's spiritual and emotional potential; and many other uses. Who knows how subtle the forces are, which can be utilized by the individual when picking up pulsations tuned into a magnet?

Dr. Bhattacharya further says "Were more known to-day of what has been forgotten in the past, it is possible that we should have a clearer view of the entire human organism constituting an electrical and magnetic field, or a magnet of a superlative kind". There is great truth in that statement. We have lost touch with so much of our heritage, and even our medical past. The only real link left is through traditional Chinese medicine. It is a great heritage, and we have been privileged to have made contact with it.

Our medicine is a medicine of the people, a caring medicine, a loving medicine, a medicine which rocks and oscillates the patient back to health. Acupuncture treatment is simple, direct and individual. It is a medicine of responsibility of the patient for himself, and this is most important. We must learn to be responsible for our own bodies, unafraid of an ache or a pain, recognizing it as a warning for which we should be grateful.

The task of the Acupuncturist is to help people to live in health and dignity. Our greatest achievement would be to work ourselves out of a job, to reach the state as in traditional China, where there was a true *health* service – where Acupuncture worked through maintaining health, while the practitioner was not paid if his charge suffered ill-health.

16　Biofeedback

A specialist is one who knows more and more about less and less –
BERNARD SHAW

. . . until he knows everything about nothing (addendum) –
SIDNEY ROSE-NEIL

Dr. ELMER GREEN[69] states 'The most significant thing that may be facilitated through training in the voluntary control of internal states, is the establishment of a Tranquility Base, not in outer space, but in inner space, on, or within, the lunar being of man.''

Biofeedback is a recent innovation to the armoury of the alternative medical practitioner, and, as such, offers much hope in the alleviation of human suffering.

It has been known for some time that a *polygraph,* an ordinary lie detector, monitors electrical changes on the skin surface. These are, in fact, forms of energy changes, there being an increased conductivity through the skin, when even the slightest amount of nervous tension is built up. Any skin energy potential increases, therefore, can be simply registered, which means that any rise in internal tensions, can also be registered. By the same token, any decrease in body tensions can, similarly, be shown. All that is needed is a machine containing an amp meter, which can be pre-set.

By having a polygraph, which is set at the body's energy resistance level at any given moment, and, by fixing electrodes to the skin surface of the hands, any change in energy potential will register on the meter. A rise or decrease in tension, however small, will register.

With the use of a polygraph, by sitting and observing the dial, one can discover which thoughts, emotions, or feelings give rise to relaxation. Using this extra understanding, the reactions can be monitored, to affect one's own bodily reactions consciously, with the goal of ultimately taking control of them.

69.　Karlins, M. and Andrews, L. M. *Biofeedback.*
　　　Warner Library, New York, U.S.A. 1973 Page 59.

Biofeedback is nature's control mechanism, each organism adjusting, every second of life, in relation to the environment, breathing, heart beats, digestion, to every movement and action of every cell in its life cycle. Therefore, the more we are able to recognize and monitor these feedbacks consciously, the greater the possibility of controlling them.

Tension, fear, and worry interfere with bodily feedback controls, and, eventually, produce such complaints as high blood pressure, asthma, migraine, arthritis, psoriasis, ulcers, and cystitis.

Recognition of abnormal deviations in energy controls provides the opportunity to rectify the balance, thus restoring health. The use of this method can do just that, easily, and within a few hours of using the machine.

Once the controls are understood, and the feelings which go with the adverse effects recognized, it is not difficult to stop producing the feelings associated with them.

The use of Biofeedback is developing in many other directions not directly associated with health, but still extremely useful. For example, it is known that many people read, by subvocalizing words as they read. This restricts reading to about a hundred and fifty words a minute. Dr. Hardyck[70] has shown that, by setting the apparatus so that, when one talks in a whisper, it registers, it becomes possible to know when one is vocalizing. With the use of Biofeedback, each time this happens, it is registered on the machine. One learns to avoid vocalization, and, in about ten hours, it can be under one's complete control, with the reading speed trebled.

Dr. Kamiya[71] has shown that Biofeedback is especially useful in the treatment of insomnia. Dr. Whatmore[72] has shown its use in psychosis, and others in the training for relaxation and meditation.

With more sophisticated apparatus, alpha, theta and delta waves are being studied, and this is leading to very useful information about the inner workings of our mental states, and how it bears on our life force. Great

70. Hardyck, C. and Petrinovich, L. *Subvocal Speech and Comprehension Level.*
     Journal of Verbal Learning 1970. No. 9. Pages 647-652.
71. Kamiya, J. *Behavioural and Physiological Concomitants of Dreaming.*
     National Institute of Health Grants 17-2116 and 17-5049. February 1962.
72. Whatmore, G. and Kohli, D. *Disponesis. A Neurological Factor in Functional Disorders.*
     Behavioral Science 1968. No. 13. Pages 102-124.

strides are also being made into the investigation of E.S.P., psychokinesis, and other paranormal activities, as well as the mysteries of altered states of consciousness. Acupuncture is closely related to Biofeedback, in that many of the mechanisms trigger off similar responses. Both Acupuncture and Biofeedback appear to monitor and bring homoeostasis to the Ch'i.

Luce and Peper[73] stated "Biofeedback promises to return us to a more holistic kind of medicine, in which the patient will acquire more responsibility for, and power over, his own health, no longer finding himself treated as a defective organ, but as a person in a context, with a life style and habits that affect his own body. Biofeedback puts the emphasis back on training, rather than the "miracle pill" or surgery, and indicates that the mind itself can be trained to do most of the things that mind-changing drugs are used for.

73.   Karlins, M. and Andrews, L. M. *Biofeedback.* Page 33.

17　Biological Transmutation

A happy mind is medicine: no better prescription exists –
CHINESE PROVERB

THE RESEARCH OF THE FRENCHMAN Louis C. Kervran[74], on biological transmutations, is of great significance to all Acupuncturists, and to everyone involved in the field of non-orthodox medicine.

For many years, it has been held by nutritional scientists that nothing is lost or gained in food metabolism – there is simply a breaking down of compounds into simpler elements, until the transformed chemical is simple enough to be absorbed by the body's cells, and rebuilt into body structure. According to this traditional outlook, nothing is ever changed; once a molecule, always a molecule, unalterable.

In order to eat safely, therefore, great margins of food elements must be consumed – extra minerals, vitamins, proteins, carbo-hydrates, oils, fats, sugars, etc. Everything must be in abundance, to be stored in the organism lest needed. It has been considered impossible for a human body, or any body of the animal kingdom, to transmute one element into another.

If we stopped for a few minutes, and pondered the fact that the human body has developed over hundreds of millions of years; that there must have been great shortages of all sorts of food elements during this time; and, in order for the body to have survived and developed, Nature must have provided mechanisms for the transmutation of elements as necessary.

Without some such facility, it seems unlikely that any animal could have developed and adjusted to the continual, and sometimes devastating, changing environment.

Kervran, by showing that elements *can* transmute (without the aid of millions of megawatts of explosive), within themselves, quietly, and without any apparent atomic explosion, will eventually bring about a medical upheaval.

74.　Abehsera, M. *Biological Transmutations*. Swan House, Binghamton, New York 1972.

The first report concerning transmutations appears to come from the French chemist Vanquelin, who, in 1799, noted a great quantity of lime being excreted by chickens. He decided to feed the chickens on oats only, and measured the amount of lime in the oats. He then measured the amount of lime excreted by the chickens, and discovered that the chickens excreted five times as much lime as was in the feedstuff.

In 1822, an English scientist called Prout showed that the amount of limestone in incubating chicks increased during incubation, and that the limestone did *not* come from the shell.

In 1831, in France, Choubard grew watercress under very controlled conditions, and showed that the plants contained elements that were not chemically explicable. Vogel, in 1844, also experimented with watercress, and provided nutriments which contained no sulphur. On re-investigation after germination, there was a definite increase in the amount of sulphur the plants contained.

During the intervening time, until Kervran began his experiments in the middle of this century, many researchers consistently showed that ecological transmutation took place, although they may not have appreciated that that was the significance, or one of the conclusions interpretable from their experiments. These experiments included Lauwes and Gilbert in the 1850's, and von Merzeele in 1875. In this century, Lakhovsky, Spindler, Branfield and others have done interesting work in similar fields.

But it was not until 1959, when Kervran first published the results of his work, that it was shown, for the first time, that molecules and atoms *can* be transformed, one to another.

The ultimate acceptance of his work must revolutionize chemistry, physics and medicine, as standardly used. It will also make *Acupuncture* more plausible and acceptable to authority.

Kervran has shown that one of our basic errors has been to attempt to explain the *whole* of nature by intransigent chemical formulae. Kervran believes that matter has a property which has been undiscovered by science, a property which is not chemical, nor within the usual accepted limits of physics, which in no way alters the present laws of chemistry or physics, but is a dimension which demands study in itself.

Kervran pointed out that, whereas *living organisms* combine nitrogen and oxygen routinely at ordinary room temperature, under laboratory conditions, electric arc temperature is necessary, and tremendous pressure.

Further, he pointed out that, as animals, we hydrolize protein in the stomach at 37 degrees in an acid medium, whereas the scientist needs a 120 degree temperature, and a concentrated acid, to achieve the same result.

It is not that Lavoisier's law is being rejected, but that other laws apply in nature, which are entirely different, which we consider to be laws of *biological transmutation*. The law of gravity is not invalidated by the fact that birds and aeroplanes fly. There are just further laws in use.

Dagognet[75] has written "The CO_2 is exhaled before the oxygen enters; more exactly, the formation of the pyruvic acid takes place without its help, or, at least, without its direct influence. We are a long way from Lavoisier and the first biochemists, who believed that respiration was combustion".

Brillouin[76] has devastated modern physio-chemistry in a few words, by showing that experiments on living animals produce different results from the experiments on dead animals. He points out that the laws of thermodynamics, as far as the degradation of energy is concerned, are reversed between working with living and working with dead matter.

In life, there is a battle to preserve life at all costs, the lesser sacrificed to the greater, and to slow down degeneration. The same material, once dead, undergoes quite a different process; degeneration becomes putrifaction, and everything moves towards degradation. The process of life is the complete opposite of the law of entropy.

At this point, it is interesting to note that all the biological laws which we have been brought up on have, perforce, been deduced from experiments on dead material.

Even the laws of elastic waves, acoustic laws, material laws, have been based upon work with non-living, inert, forms. The discoveries are excellent, when applied to understanding or affecting inorganic matter, but have little or no application to living organisms.

75.   Dagognet L. *Methodes et Doctrines dans l'Oeuvre de Parteur*. Edit. PUF 1967.
76.   Brillouin, L. *Vie, Matiere et Observations*. Edit. A. Michel, Paris 1959.

Kervran pointed out that the living and dead are like the front and the back. He pointed out the laws of yin and yang. The front and back are inseparable, yet complementary, a unique principle with two faces. Kervran says: "To reject biological transmutations *a priori* in the name of nuclear physics, a science based upon observation of dead matter, is to evince an ignorance of this duality (yin and yang) which exists in all aspects of physics". Kervran concluded from his researches that biological transmutations are not of a chemical order, but go deeply into the atom. Chemistry, as we know it, is the final stage of the molecular arrangement. Nature moves particles from one atom to another, not only hydrogen and oxygen, but even carbon and lithium. The nuclei of light elements are different from those of the heavy elements. Biological phenomena are different from the atomic fission accepted by physics. The principle generally outlined by Kervran show that there are properties of matter not yet understood by orthodox physics.

An interesting experiment conducted by Kervran on a team of workers who were drilling in the Sahara desert, showed that, when it was very hot, a great deal of potassium was exceted via the skin. Due to taking quantities of sea-salt, the men were able to work for long periods unprotected and unshaded from the sun, even working on metallic plates. The experiment was carried out under strict conditions over six months. Yet, in spite of long and protracted checking, it was found that much less salt was excreted than was ingested, and far more potassium than could have been stored in the body. There seemed only one possible explanation – the sea-salt must have been transformed into potassium.

In another experiment, using terrestrial and marine iguana, Kervran showed that up to a hundred and ninety times more potassium was excreted than was to be found in the blood plasma of the animals. It was found that, when sodium chloride was added to the cesspool, it produced an increase in the *potassium* excretion, but none in the sodium excretion.

Von Merzeele[77] showed that seeds, without any supply of calcium, had an increase in the calcium found in the plants thirty days after germination. After he had proved this phenomenon repeatedly, against great opposition,

77.   Von Merzeele. Brochures published in 1875 and 1883 by Mermann Peters, Berlin.

no logical explanation could be offered. Only now, in accordance with Kervran's biological transmutation concept, can it be understood.

Another interesting experiment which Kervran carried out was to prove that potassium could be transformed into calcium. Hens were kept in a coop on clay soil, with very little limestone. When the supply of limestone within the soil was exhausted, it became immediately apparent, as the shells became very thin. *Mica* was then given to the hens, who consumed it with vigour. By the very next day, normal egg shells were being produced, showing that the silicate of potassium contained in the mica, had been transformed into the necessary calcium.

It is an accepted phenomenon that a hatched chicken has four times more calcium in its bones than is contained in the yolk and white of the egg combined. Some researchers have attempted to claim that the calcium comes from the shell, but this has not been substantiated. The same phenomenon occurs with fish, where there is no shell, even with fresh-water fish, where there is almost no calcium!

According to Kervran, strange things happen when fruit is dried, as large amounts of many elements vanish. He showed that transmutations take place in potassium, sodium, calcium, silicon, magnesium, phosphorus, nitrogen, sulphur, chlorine, manganese, iron, and other elements.

Kervran stated that biological mutation takes place regularly in plants. For farmers who have continued to produce organically, there is no question. For example, sulphur is continually found in oat crops which grow in clay soil, which is impermeable.

Fertilizers are sold in massive quantities to replace used up nitrogen, potassium, and sodium, yet the plants manage, unaided, to replace all the *other* elements extracted from the earth each year, in time for the next year's crop. Where do they come from?

Traditionally, it has been believed that allowing the soil to lie fallow permitted the elements which have become exhausted to reappear. The assumption for this has been that the fresh elements are brought by dust, winds, animals and migration through the soil, yet no evidence has been presented for this contention. In fact, hundreds of acres of land may be being cultivated, farm by farm, in similar rotation, all using similar elements.

127

18 Body Clocks, Cycles, etc.

A full conception of the science will never be achieved by the knowledge of only part of it – CHARAKA

FOR THOUSANDS OF YEARS it has been taught in Acupuncture that the body has a series of rhythms, forms of expanding and contracting, tension and relaxation, opening and closing, high energy and low energy, yin and yang, coming and going. The Chinese proverb applies well to Acupuncture 'All that has a back has a front, the broader the back the broader the front'.

The acupuncture clock chart has been one of the concepts most difficult for the orthodox doctor to accept. Even some Acupuncturists, with an orthodox training in medicine, have rejected the acupuncture clock principle. Yet modern science is coming more and more around to the idea that universal clocks, world clocks and body clocks are legion. In life, it has always been accepted that such clocks exist. Do we not need sleep every night? Is there not a rhythm in our toilet habits, our eating habits? Is menstruation not a regular occurrence? These clocks are not associated with body chemistry, but with energy, electro-magnetic forces, static-electrical forces, gravity. In fact, they operate in spite of body chemistry, rather than because of it.

It is my belief that Acupuncture is closely associated with such universal rhythms, and good Acupuncture puts the person back in rhythm with his natural clocks. This resonance vibrates through the organism, and hums the body back to health, just as a gyroscope, put back in tune with its correct vibrations, forces out the incorrect vibration. Ripples go through water in ever-widening circles; these vibrations tune into the natural rhythm of the atom, and rectify imbalance, thereby bringing about vibrant health. It is these resonances which we tune into, at the Chinese pulses.

Biological and cosmic rhythms are basic to life – to animals, and to plants, and to every molecule and atom. Does not each life atom always revolve in the same precise formation, does not the earth consistently move around the sun; and the moon around the earth? Do we not breathe with a rhythm, and the blood circulate to the rhythm of the heart? Without rhythm, the universe could not exist for one millionth of a second.

Can the atom control the rhythm, if it is itself a part of it? Can the atom control that which surrounds it? Only by influencing outgoing rippling vibrations from its centre. Then what is the ripple? The resonance? The vibration? The radiation? Certainly, it is not the atom, because, if it were, it would remain within the atom. Its vibration would be part of it, until it was picked up by the next atom, would then become part of the next atom, and so on, in which case, there could be no space between the atoms, and all atoms would become one. Maybe all *is* one, and, in becoming one, we are all separate. This is pure Zen.

Present researchers[78] seem to indicate that there are four basic rhythms — one related to the moon turning on its axis, the second to the earth turning on its axis, the third to the passage of the moon around the earth, and the fourth the earth moving around the sun. From these rhythms come others, related to hot and cold, light and dark, ebb and flow of the tides, etc.

Until recently, the clock best known to man was the earth clock, the time it takes for the earth to turn on its axis, the sidereal day, twenty-three hours and fifty-six minutes. But, recently, scientists have discovered that this movement varies, and now the atomic clock has replaced the earth clock. The variation in the earth's rotation comes from the influence of cosmic forces, gravitational pushes and pulls. If these forces influence the movement of the earth, even for only fractions of a second, how much more influence must they have on man?

Adderly and Bowen[79] have found that most rainfall falls immediately before a new and a full moon.

The sun is in permanent effervescence, expanding and contracting burning gas. These boiling gases explode, and can be seen as so-called 'sun-spots'. The effects of these sun-spots reach the earth, and affect our weather, our radios, and our bodies. Our own life and activities must also be affected and influenced by them. Cyclones (rain), and anti-cyclones (warm), are

78. Luce, G. G. *Body Time*. Maurice Temple Smith, London, England 1971.
79. Adderley, E. E. *Lunar Component in Precipitation Date*.
     Science 1962. No. 137. Page 749.

known to be caused by such eruptions. This was discovered in Germany by Berg, and the Austrian scientiest, Hanzlik[78].

Tree rings indicate the age of the tree. These rings vary in thickness, depending upon the tree's nourishment during that year, and on the climatic conditions. By looking at tree rings, it is possible to reconstruct the weather of bygone days for thousands of years. In Arizona, Professor Douglas studied tree rings, and discovered that it followed precisely the rhythm of recorded *sun* activity, particularly the rhythm of the eleven-year sunspot pattern, first observed by a man named Acabe in 1840. During great sun activation, there is heavy rainfall, causing wide rings, and, during more limited sun-spot activity, there is less rainfall, and resultant narrower rings. It has been recorded in France that the best Burgundy wines have been produced where there has been the most sun-spot activity, and therefore the most rain. The same phenomenon has been observed with Rhine wines, produced over the last two hundred years.

Also, varves, the thin layers of mud laid down in the bottom of lakes, have been studied by Edward Dewey[78]. He discovered that, in the same way as the trees, varve layers can be distinguished, year by year, and they vary in thickness. In a warm year, where there is more melting of ice, and therefore more deposits reach the lake bottoms, the varves are thicker. With these new diagnostic tools, it has become possible to measure the average temperature over many thousands of years. Any regularity of varve thickness means a weather cycle, and it can be recognized that, for hundreds of thousands of years, there has been a definite cycle of weather, which is approximately our eleven-year cycle. Dr. Piccardi[80], of the Institute of Physical Chemistry in Florence, states that this has been so for *hundreds of millions of years*.

Then, beyond the eleven-year cycle, Wolf, a Swiss astronomer, has shown another cycle, which is between eighty and a hundred years, which is now called the secular rhythm. During this period, the sun's activity increases for about one half of the time, about forty years, and decreases for the other half. The cycle is then repeated. This is confirmed in the lake bottom varves.

78.   Luce, G.G. *Body Time*. Maurice Temple Smith, London, England 1971.
80.   Piccardi, G. *Expose Introductif*. Presses Academiques Europeennes, Brussels 1969.

This theory has been re-inforced by the discoveries of a German botanist, Schnelle[81]. He studied the appearance of snowdrops between 1870 and 1950, in Frankfurt. He noted that the average first-flowering was February 23rd. Using this as his base line, he estimated the flowering before and after the base date, and produced a curve which showed the same eighty-year cycle. Mironovitch[78], a French meteorologist, took this research even further, and showed that, when the snowdrops were early, there was low sun-spot activity, and, when they were late, there was great solar activity, again within the eighty-year cycle. He concluded that the solar activity influenced the winds, which influenced the plants, also relating the influence of increased sun activity to earthquake patterns.

Zhan Ze-Zia, a Soviet scientist, studied typhoons in China, and found that there was a direct correlation between solar activity within the eighty-year cycle and the number of typhoons, which increased with the increase of sun activity.

With so much inter-relationship throughout Nature, it is not surprising to realize that cyclic influences are at work in our every-day life and health.

For example, it is interesting to note that disease symptoms are not distributed evenly around the clock, that more women go into labour and more coronary attacks occur during the night and early morning than during the day.

According to Sancorious, a seventeenth century doctor, ordinary healthy people vary in weight by as as much as two pounds over a monthly cycle. Hamburger[78], a Danish endocrinologist, discovered a monthly urinary cycle as well as a daily one.

Bohlen[78], of Wisconsin University, discovered that body temperature and potassium excretion followed a twenty-four hour rhythm, which extends to a whole year, with as much as ten times the calcium being excreted in the winter compared with the summer.

Dr. Haus and Dr. Hamburg discovered a yearly cycle in mice, in regard to their blood levels in adrenal hormones, and in cortisone. These animals

78.   Luce G.G. *Body Time*.
81.   Schnelle, F. *Hundert Jahre*. Meteorol. Rundschau 1950. No. 7.
82.   Mironovitch, V. *Abhand Lungen*. Meteorol. Rundschau 1969. No. 9. Page 3.

were kept in controlled environments, with standardized lighting, in order to exclude ordinary environmental factors. The experiment showed that the mice were influenced by forces beyond the environmental conditions.

In another experiment, bees were trained to consume sugar-water at a certain time. They were then taken from France to the United States. They went to collect their sugar-water at the correct time for *France,* not for the United States, showing that light or dark were not their measure, but more subtle forces. We take many body rhythms for granted, for example the heart and pulse sixty to eighty beats a minute.

Dr. Hildebrandt[78], of Marburg University, substantiated what the Yellow Emperor taught thousands of years ago, that the relationship between the heart beat and the pulse should be in the ratio of four to one.

If we go on a jet trip across the world, we are soon aware of our body rhythms. This has been learned at great cost to many international companies, who have found that their executives should not make major decisions until they have adjusted to the new environment, and re-orientated the body clocks.

Even our breathing is uneven, particularly notable when we have a cold, because we normally breath- first with one nostril, then with the other. Yogis have known this for hundreds of years. In good health, we breathe through each nostril, with an alternate cycle of about three hours.

There is no doubt that, although many rhythms may be internally controlled, there are cosmic influences as well. We have not only adjusted to the cosmic clocks to produce our own internal rhythms, but we are also ceaselessly influenced by cosmic rhythms.

In Acupuncture, we use these life forces for the benefit of the patient. We influence the forces, directing, re-aligning, balancing, stimulating and sedating them. By normalizing these life forces, the chemistry of the body is influenced, the molecules and atoms are set on the right road again, health and vitality pulse through the body.

Time structure is important in old age, and it is now considered that each cell in the organism can reproduce only a certain number of times, and one's life span is directly related to the number of reproductions of cells.

78.   Luce G.G. *Body Time.*

It would appear that the circadian rhythm, the twenty-four hour rhythm, would tend to change with advancing age, if it were connected directly to the molecular atomic structure of the organism; in other words, if the rhythm were chemically controlled rather than cosmically controlled.

Dr. Montalbetti, in Milan, investigated seventeen different hydro-cortico-steroids found in the urine of the aged. He discovered that, where there was a disturbance, it was due to sleep or urinary-tract problems, and that there was always basically the normal circadian rhythm.

Dr. Kreiger[78], in New York, in a similar experiment, had a comparable result. During the day, our temperature rises and falls in a controlled cycle. In the afternoon and early evening, when our temperature is at its highest, we are usually more energetic.

But, nowadays, our lives are so full of artificiality, that we hardly, if at all, notice the many changes which take place within our bodies.

A cat, on the other hand, will abide by its body functions and desires, working closely with its biological clocks, resting, eating, playing, running, hunting, sleeping, but always in an obviously relaxed harmony within itself.

Man in our present society, with its push and struggle, has lost much of his rapport with nature. Our bodies, whether we appreciate it or not, are in a state of constant change and flux.

We may not be aware of many of these changes, but, in spite of that, we behave differently at different times of the day; and why not, because we are almost a different being, as far as our body rhythms are concerned.

In spite of the evidence to the contrary, many scientists have stuck to the concept that these rhythms are internally controlled, and of a chemical nature. For example, Dr, Bunning[78], of Berlin, claimed that all seeds held a genetically-controlled memory, the memory-clock to an oscillating in-built physico system which continues, independent of any rhythmic alterations in the organism's environment.

These scientists believe that the time factor for these cycles are inherited, and only bear a cosmic relationship with natural geophysical rhythms due to the millions of years of adaptation through evolution.

78.   Luce, G.G. *Body Time.*

To my mind, this theory is closely linked to the Mendalian theory of evolution, held by many orthodox scientists, which keeps the organism isolated from the environment, even after millions of years, and only allows for adaptation as a continuing accident of trial and error. But the theory does not allow for cosmic links, for inherited learning, or for evolution as a joint effort. The theory no longer fits all known facts, and much work has been done to demonstrate the cosmic influence on living matter.

At Yale, Dr. Burr[83] experimented with trees, and studied their electrical potential. By drilling two holes in a tree, and inserting the ends of a piece of wire, he was able to test the current passing through the wire, produced by the tree. He found that, not only did the voltage vary, but the current flowed one way, and then the other. His experiment showed that the phase of the moon altered the electrical potential, and, further, sun-spot activity had a direct bearing on the voltage and current flow. How or why this voltage change was taking place, or why the current changed direction, has not been explained. It seems obvious, however, that the tree tunes in to cosmic electrical or magnetic forces.

Could it be that there is some form of explanation here, as to why there is a yin and yang force in the body, and why some of the meridians are yang and some yin, and why they are more forceful at certain times than at others? It could be that, towards the early afternoon, as the body swings into greater activity, its overall tuning is more towards yang, and, as late night comes, the organism swings into yin. The individual meridians may still retain their yin or yang activity, but the overall pattern of the body may change from yin to yang, and from yang to yin, as the lunar day passes its influences through us.

One thing is certain, that these and the many other phenomena being discussed in this paper, cannot be understood in terms of chemistry alone.

Stcherbinovsky, a Russian entomologist, investigated the migration of locusts for forty years throughout the world. He found a direct relationship between the location of the insects and the eleven-year sunspot cycle of the sun. Dejavin, another Russian, noted a similar phenomenon, with the death and reproduction rate of sturgeon.

83.   Burr, H. S. (Author of many works) *Diurnal Potentials in Maple Tree.*

The age of coral flabellum is known by its striations, and, while it is simple to explain a yearly striation, it is not so easy to explain monthly and daily ones. An explanation was put forward that it is due to the tides, to light, and to the lunar cycle generally. Unfortunately for this theory, some varieties of this coral live at a very great depth, where there is neither tide nor light, but the striations still occur.

In the *American Scientist,* Dr. Brown[78] explained an experiment in which he used potatoes and carrots. He measured the quantity of oxygen which was released by these tubers. He found that there was a significant oxygen-consumption change, corresponding to weather changes, except that it happened two days *before* the weather change. He then did similar experiments with oysters, crabs, salamanders, seaweed and rats, and all showed the same results.

The British astronomers Leaton, Malin and Finch[84] discovered that animals are able to react, and follow solar and lunar vibrational rhythms. Brown calculated from these experiments, that an animal has an inbuilt mechanism to tune into the geophysical oscillations, a form of 'living magnetometer'. Surely, this may be the way birds migrate, and E.S.P. may work, picking up feelings, words and ideas from other animals. We tune in, through our bodies, with others and the cosmos.

Many rhythms we work with unconsciously, others we block by our consciousness, our determination to be physical, materialistic, to accept only that which we can see, slowly ruining our inbuilt ability to use these cosmic vibrations, even our ability to pick them up.

Children are always using them, often knowing what a parent is thinking. When an adult is sad, however well he may cover it up, an uncanny intuition, or is it inherited ability to know our feelings, to sense danger, to pick up our oscillation, the child asks "What is the matter?" "Nothing" answers the parent, unwilling to burden a little child with what is wrong, at the moment, in his adult world. The child naturally believes the parent, and so the mechanism becomes slowly discouraged, and nearly lost. When we reach

78.   Luce, G.G. *Body Time.*
84.   *Yale Journal of Biology and Medicine.* 1945. No. 17. Page 727.
      Leaton, Malin and Finch *The Solar and Luni-Solar Variations of the Geomagnetic Field.*
      Observatory Bulletin of Great Britain 1962. No. 53. Page 273.

adulthood ourselves, our E.S.P. is at a low ebb; we still get hunches, but usually put them down to coincidence.

Dr. Brown did further experiments with a form of slug, called the nassarius. These molluscs were placed in a coral with some water, with only a small exit aperture, so small that only one animal could pass through at a time. 33,000 nassarius were checked. At certain times of the day, they left in one direction, which slowly changed over the period of the day. After further research, it was shown that this changing orientation of direction exactly related to the phases of the moon, coinciding with the change of terrestrial magnetism.

Further experiments, with fresh water flatworms, produced similar results. As the new moon came, the flat-worm turned as much as ten degrees north, and, at the full moon, it changed its direction to ten degrees in the opposite direction.

At the University of Illinois, Dr. Palmer[85] observed 7,000 volvox, a tiny organism less than a millimetre long, moving in similar rhythms.

Dr. Becker, in Germany, has shown that flies do not land at random, but keep to certain magnetic lines, as if they were more comfortable, or possibly recharged with energy if working, flying and landing in certain directions.

Dr. Koig, of Munich, has demonstrated that low energy long-waves, on only one to ten Hertz, up to over a hundred thousand miles long, can influence the sprouting of wheat and the activity and growth of bacteria and insects. The longer the wave, the greater its penetration power, because of its minute amptitude. The wave is not stopped by any atom, and yet living matter can sense, use, and be influenced by these energy vibrations.

Gravitation, also, must have an influence on every living tissue; nothing can escape. It is so slight, so gentle, that it cannot be felt as such, and yet it pulls everything back to earth.

The earth's magnetic pull is so small, only four-tenths of a gauss, and yet its importance is beyond dispute. Without gravitation, there would be no life, without the sun's gravitation, the earth would be spinning endlessly, and lost in space. The moon's pull causes tides, in a similar way to the oceans.

85.   Palmer, J. D. *Organismic Spatial Orientation in Weak Magnetic Fields.*
       Nature 1963. No. 198 Page 1061.

Why cannot it also affect our blood stream, our interstitial liquids, our plasma and lymph?

If we think in terms of Darwin's law of the survival of the fittest, adapt or perish, it may well be that, over hundreds of millions of years, all living things adapted to changing climate by the day, and by the season, recognizing before the event that these changes are about take place, tuning into and acting upon cosmic vibrations, just as birds move across the world for their summer vacation.

Dr. Brown takes an interesting stand-point, by claiming that internal physical-chemical clocks are not needed at all, as all living things are able to tune into the cosmic clocks. Dr. Brown includes magnetism, static electrical fields, gravitation, and all other forms of radiation which influence organisms. Further, he claims that only experiments in space can isolate man from his cosmic environment, and from his much-used life cycles.

Many animals show both a lunar and a solar cycle. For example, fiddler crabs show a repeated colour change, getting darker and lighter each day, even if they are kept in complete isolation. This colour change is in keeping with the solar cycle, but, on the other hand, their work-activity cycle is in rhythm with the lunar cycle, 24.8 hours, as against the twenty-four hour solar cycle.

That we receive information from some form of cosmic signal, has indirectly been believed by every farmer from time immemorial. The ancient Greeks knew that it was best to plant certain crops together, and keep others away from each other. Some lived in harmony, while others appeared to be out of tune. Further, they always planted crops in phase with the moon, keeping exactly the same time for certain crops. They also always planted North to South. This latter way of planting is still accepted by many so-called backward nations. As mentioned before, many people have noticed that they sleep better head North and feet South. It seems to recharge them.

The action of birds indicate a hot or a long summer, or a hard or mild winter; fiddler crabs are said to hide in inland burrows two days before a hurricane.

Canadian foresters predict snow by the elk, which will go to shelter two days before the snow starts.

Without sleep, man becomes ill and would die; with reduced sleep, he is irritable, unable to work well, cannot concentrate. In encephalitis, the patient exchanges night for day, and it is, in fact, a sign of that illness. Narcolepsy is another sleep illness. Why do we need sleep? Can it be that the body chemistry needs a rest? Why? To cleanse itself, get rid of impurities? These explanations are not logical, for Nature could easily have developed methods to cleanse the cells as they work, indeed they do.

There is no evidence that the cells need to be cleansed by sleep, that cellular toxins collect during wakefulness, to be discharged during the night. Body excretion takes place day *and* night.

It would seem more reasonable to assume that a recharging is needed, of some forms of energy; the body needing to retune to the cosmos, to re-oscillate itself, to re-align its centre, to find itself cosmically, to listen to the sound of its 'one hand clapping'. The circadian rhythm expresses itself, in spite of all pressures that the scientists may put upon it.

Dr Richter[78], of John Hopkins University, Baltimore, attempted to alter the twenty-four hour rhythms of rats. They were given shocks, drugs, exposed to freezing, had their hearts stopped, portions of the brain removed, and blinded. But the animals still showed their twenty-four hour circadian rhythm.

Professor Adolph Smith[86], of Sir George Williams University, Montreal, has been interested in Acupuncture for some years, and particularly in whether adenosine triphosphate (A.T.P.), the body's basic chemical-energy unit, is related to Acupuncture. It is interesting to note that the production and break-down of A.T.P. has been shown to be rhythmic.

Dr. Pittendrigh[87], in the United States, has been able to measure A.T.P. break-down in the liver of hampsters. In fact, what happens is that, when a cell requires chemical energy, the water contained in the cell breaks down the chemical bonding of the A.T.P., which is hydrolysis. When this happens, a phosphate is stripped from the A.T.P. – forming adenosine-ei-phosphate (A.D.P.), which releases chemical-energy.

78.   Luce G.G. *Body Time.*
86.   Smith, Professor A. Private paper to the author 1971.
87.   Pittendrigh, C.S., V.G. *Daily Rhythms as Coupled Oscillator Systems.*
     Washington 1959.

The team raised these hamsters in a false environment of twelve day and twelve night hours. As they work nocturnally, they were, of course, most active during the dark period. The livers were taken from the animals and centrifuged, thus separating the A.T.P. and A.D.P. from the rest of its tissue. It was found that more A.T.P. was being broken down at night than during the day, allowing the animal to be more active during its nocturnal period. As the animals had been kept under false conditions, the experiment showed that the A.T.P. breakdown was not controlled by internal body clocks, but by *external* influences.

Light, without doubt, plays an important part in our physiology. Under the direction of Dr. Reinberg[88], of Paris, a young woman went underground for eighty-eight days, in isolation. It was found that, underground, her normal twenty-four cycle changed to 24.6 hours, a statistical difference. During her normal life, her menstrual cycle was twenty-nine days. While underground, her menstrual cycle changed to 25.7 days. On returning to normal life, the cycle returned to its former twenty-nine days. This experiment led Dr. Reinberg into investigating forms of light as an influence on menstruation. A study of six hundred girls in Germany showed that menarche started most frequently in the winter. A further study in Prague produced a similar result. It appears that dim light, or the lack of long periods of light, acts as stimulus to the menstrual cycle. Blind girls reach menarche before seeing girls.

It is, further, interesting to note that, when several females live together for a while, their menses tune in, and eventually start and finish at approximately the same time. This is not something which can be explained by body chemistry. It seems that light therapy and colour therapy may have a great deal to offer in the not too distant future, and the many practitioners who have been practising it, may soon have some very influential scientific allies.

Professor Kim Bong Han, the research worker at Pyang Yang University of North Korea, showed experimentally that light influenced the energy potential at the acupoints, there being a substantial reduction of body activity, energy and well-being when the points were deprived of light.

88.   Reinberg, A. and Ghata, J. *Biological Rhythms and Cycles.* Paris University Press 1957.

Dr. Everett and Dr. Sawyer[78], of Duke University, showed that rats kept under constant light went into estrus. Rats, put into darkness some hours before the critical time, will not ovulate. Male hamsters' gonads atrophy if the animal is deprived of light. A room without light soon takes on a strange and nasty smell. Plants cannot grow without light, unless they are a certain type of fungus such as a mushroom. We generally think in terms of the solar day of twenty-four hours when considering menstruation, but the lunar day may exert more of an influence in some people, lasting twenty-three hours and fifty minutes, or the synovial month lasting 29.5 days. Once again, every month of the 29.5 days, the sun and the moon rise and set at the same time. This cycle may have a great deal to do with many organic functions.

There is no doubt that light is very complex, as far as the living world is concerned, and, medically, important. During our everyday life, we go about, ill-concerned about the intensity of light, and of the colours around us, yet colour-intensity and light-intensity influence menstruation, maturation and other organic functions. Many experiments have been carried out in the Max-Planck subterranean apartments which have proved that man in influenced by magnetic electro-fields, that his cycles change when these fields are shielded. False electro-fields were introduced into the laboratory, up to a thousand times stronger than the earth's fields. The life-cycle rhythms shortened and were disturbed.

However, it should be appreciated that the life-energy circadian rhythms have not been successfully altered for long periods of time. All animals, finally, appear to pick up the correct influences around them, and use them for the benefit of their own existence. There is still no evidence that any animal or plant can adapt to a non-material circadian cycle. Nature pulsates, and pulsates ceaselessly, and, in the end, wins, even if, ultimately, it means destroying a whole species, as it surely will do with man if he continues to destroy his cosmic environment. One thing is certain. Acupuncture is the most natural of treatments, and fits perfectly into the natural cycles of Nature, using them, and not hindering or destroying them.

78. Luce G.G. *Body Time.*

Conclusion

IT IS APPARENT that much of the present day research into the non-orthodox sciences ties in well with acupuncture energy researches. These consistently point to an underlying unity, and Acupuncture can only be strengthened by the continuing stream of evidence.

Should this work have stimulated the reader's interest into believing, or even considering, that Acupuncture will, finally, be explained in terms of energy rather than chemistry, then it has been well worth the effort.

References

1. Rhyme, Wilhelm den. *Amoenitatum Exoticarum*, 1712. British Museum, North Library.
2. Veith, Ilza. *The Yellow Emperor's Classic of Internal Medicine.*
    Williams and Wilkins Company, Baltimore, U.S.A., 1949. Page 149.
3. Ibid. Page 97.
4. Ibid. Page 150.
5. Ibid. Page 150.
6. Ibid. Page 152.
7. Ibid. Page 168.
8. Confucius. *The Book of Rites.*
9. Russell, Bertrand. *History of Western Philosophy.*
10. Bachmann, Gerhard, Professor, Dr. Medicine. *Die Akupunktur eine Ordnungstherapie.*
    Karl Haug Verlas, Ulm-Donau. Germany, 1959.
11. Rusetzky, J.J., Professor. *The Chinese Method of Therapeutic Needling.*
    Tartar Publication, 1950.
12. Bachmann, Gerhard, Professor, Dr. Medicine. *Basic Information on Acupuncture.*
    Lecture at Congress of Reflex Therapy. Gorki, U.S.S.R. May 1960.
13. Kervran, Dr. Louis C. *Biological Transmutations.* Swan House, Binghamton, N.Y. 1972.
14. Wheaton, John. Lecture to Acupuncture Congress, 1972.
15. Wall, Professor Pat. *New Scientist* 20 July, 1972.
16. Seminar on Acupuncture at University of Rotterdam Medical School 12 October 1972.
17. Panati, Charles. *The Geller Papers.* Houghton Mifflin, Boston, U.S.A. 1976
18. Kervran, Dr. Louis. Ibid.
19. Ostrander and Schroeder. *Psychic Discoveries Behind the Iron Curtain.*
    Bantam Books. Prentice Hall, New Jersey, U.S.A. 1970. Page 366.
20. Ostrander and Schroeder. Ibid. Page 368.
21. Ostrander and Schroeder. Ibid. Page 374.
22. Krishnamurti, J. *The First and Last Freedom* (and other works).
    Victor Gollancz, London, 1972.
23. *Acupuncture Anaesthesia.* Foreign Language Press, Peking 1972. Page 26.
24. *Which* Magazine, London 1972.
25. *Irish Medical Times* 16 June 1972
26. Manaka and Urquhart. *The Layman's Guide to Acupuncture.*
    Wetherhill, New York, U.S.A. 1972. Page 26.
27. Manaka and Tani. *Electrical Studies on the Skin Surface of the Human Body.*
    Odswara, Japan October 1969.
28. *Journal of Paraphysics* Volume 6 No. 2 1972. Downtown, Wiltshire: England. Page 82.
29. Ostrander and Schroeder. Ibid. Page 229.

30. Walter Thompson and Peter Gilhead. Members of the British Acupuncture Association.

31. Ostrander and Schroeder. Ibid. Many referernces.

32. Sergeyev Shushkev and Gryaznukkir. *Journal of Paraphysics*
    Volume 6 No. 1 1972. Downtown, Wiltshire, England.

33. Ostrander and Schroeder. Ibid. Page 202

34. Kozyrev, Nikolai *An Unexplored World* Soviet Life. November 1965.

35. Koryrev, Nikolai *Possibility of Experimental Study of the Properties of Time.*
    Joint publications, Research Service, Department of Commerce, U.S.A. 6 May 1968.

36. Reich, Wilhelm *Cosmic Superimposition.* Orgone Institute Press, Maine, U.S.A. 1951.

37. Bong Han, Professor Kim *On the Kyungrak System.* Pyongyang, Korea 1964.

38. The Kyoto Pain Control Institute, 280 Shimizucho Takatsuji Kawaramachi, Shimogyo,
    Kyoto, Japan.

39. Lakhovsky, G. *The Secret of Life.* True Healthy Publishing Co., Rustington, Sussex,
    England 1973. Heinemann 1933.

40. Eeman, L.S. *Cooperative Healing.* Frederick Muller, London W.C.1, England 1947.

41. Kilner, Walter *The Kirlian Aura.* New York. University Books 1965.

42. Kushi, Michio. Founder East West Foundation, 62, Buckminster Road, Boston, U.S.A.

43. Bong Han, Professor Kim *Kyungrak System and Theory of Sanal.*
    Medical Science Press, Pyongyang, Korea 1965.

44. Reich, Wilhelm *Ether, God and Devil.* Orgone Institute Press, Maine, U.S.A. 1949.

45. Reich, Wilhelm *Character Analysis.* Moonday Press U.S.A.

46. Todaro, G. and Huebner, R. *The Viral Oncogen Hypothesis - New Evidence.*
    Proc. Nat. Acad. Sci. (U.S.A.) 69 1009 (1972).

47. Temin, H.M. *The R.N.A. Tumor Viruses, Background and Foreground.*
    Proc. Nat. Acad. Sci. (U.S.A.) 69 1016 (1972).

48. Reich, Wilhelm *The Cancer Biopathy.* Moonday Press, U.S.A.

49. Laszlo, E. *Introduction to Systems Philosophy.* New York, Gordon and Breach 1972.

50. Fuller, R.B. *Intuition.* New York. Doubleday and Co., 1972.

51. Moss, T. and Johnson K. *Radiation Field Photography.* Psychic 1972. Pages 50-54.

52. Moss, T. *Searching for Psi* Psychic 1971 - 2. Pages 40-44.

53. Krippner, S. and Rubin, D. *The Kirlian Aura.* Anchor Books, New York 1974.

54. Inyushin, V.M. *On the Biological Essence of the Kirlian Effect.*
    Alma-Ata, Kazakj, U.S.S.R. Kazakj University 1968

55. Adamenko, V.G. *Electrodynamics of Living Systems.* Journal of Paraphysics,
    Volume 4, No. 4, 1970. Downtown, Wiltshire, England. Pages 113-120.

56. Press, A.S. *The Role of Electromagnetic Fields in Vital Processes.* Biofizika 1964, Gilz.

57. Lakatos, I., Meeting of the Aristotelian Society. 21 Bedford Square,
    London W.C.1, England October 1968.

58. Tiller, Professor W. *The Kirlian Aura.* Stamford University, U.S.A. 1973.

59. Davis, R.A. and Rawls, W.C. *Magnetism and its Effect on the Living System.*
    Exposition Press, Hicksville, NVEW York 1974.

60. Davis and Bhattacharya *Magnet and Magnetic Fields.* Mukhopodhyay, Calcutta 1970.

61. Fuzimoto, S. *The Magnetic Band.* "Aimante." Internal Dept. Red Cross Hospital, Kyoto, Japan 1963.
     Nakagawa and others *Biological Effects of Magnetic Fields* Dept. of Int. Med., Isuza Hospital, Tokyo, Japan 1963.

62. Ewart, A.J. *On the Physics and Physiology of Protoplasmic Streaming in Plants.* Clarendon Press 1903.

63. Jennison, M.W. *Journal of Bacteriology.* 1937 Volume 33, Pages 15-16.

64. Nakagawa *Journal of Japanese Society of Internal Medicine.* 1958 Volume 47, No. 1, Page 74.

65. Sswastin, P.W. *Planta.* 11, Pages 683-720 1930.

66. Lenzi, M. *Strahlentherapie.* 1940 67, Pages 219-250.

67. Hansen, K.M. *Acta Medica Scandinavica.* 1938 97, Pages 339-364.

68. Nanbu, Japanese Tobata National Railway Hospital 1960.

69. Karlins, M. and Andrews, L.M. *Biofeedback.* Warner Library, New York, U.S.A. 1973. Page 59.

70. Hardyck, C. and Petrinovich, L. *Subvocal Speech and Comprehension Level.* Journal of Verbal Learning 1970, No. 9. Page 647-652.

71. Kamiya, J. *Behavioral and Physiological Concomitants of Dreaming.* National Institute of Health Grants 17-2116 and 17-5049 February 1962.

72. Whatmore, G. and Kohli, D. *Disponesis. A Neurological Factor in Functional Disorders.* Behavioral Science 1968 No. 13, Pages 102-124.

73. *Biofeedback.* Ibid. Page 33.

74. Abehsera, M. *Biological Transmutations.* Swan House, Binghamton, New York 1972.

75. Dagognet L. *Methodes et Doctrines dans l'Oeuvre de Parteur.* Edit PUF 1967.

76. Brillouin, L. *Vie, Matiere et Observations.* Edit. A. Michel, Paris 1959.

77. Von Merzeele, Brochures published in 1875 and 1883 by Mermann Peters, Berlin.

78. Luce, G.G. *Body Time.* Maurice Temple Smith, London, England 1971.

79. Adderley, E.E. and Bowen, E.G. *Lunar Component in Precipitation Date.*
     Science 1962 No. 137, Page 749.

80. Piccardi, G. *Expose Introductif.* Presses Academiques Europeennes, Brussels 1969.

81. Schnelle, F. *Hundert Jahre.* Meteorol. Rundschau 1950. No. 7.

82. Mironovitch, V. *Abhand Lungen.* Meteorol. Rundschau 1960. No. 9, Page 3.

83. Burr, H.S. (Author of many works) *Diurnal Potentials in the Maple Tree.*

84. *Yale Journal of Biology and Medicine.* 1945. No. 17, Page 727.
     Leaton, Malin and Finch *The Solar and Luni-Solar Variations of the Geomagnetic Field.* Observatory Bulletin of Great Britain 1962. No. 53, Page 273.

85. Palmer, J.D. *Organismic Spatial Orientation in Weak Magnetic Fields.*
     Nature 1963. No. 198, Page 1061.

86. Smith, Professor A. Private paper to the author 1971.

87. Pittendrigh, C.S. and Bruce, V.G. *Daily Rhythms as Coupled Oscillator Systems.* Washington 1959.

88. Reinberg, A. and Ghata, J. *Biological Rhythms and Cycles.* Paris University Press 1957.

Basic Premises and Pertinent Questions

There are no miracles, only unknown laws – Saint Augustine (41)
Atoms can alter their structure, become other elements – Kervran

There is nothing random in Nature. (41)

Structural integrity is fundamental, the whole being more than the sum of its parts. (41) Survival of the organism is the deciding factor. (41) The lesser subordinates its needs to the greater. (41)

Function controls structure through a process of priority. (69) Everything in the body functions and it is the function which counts. (69)

Nature is controlled by energy, not chemistry. (36)

Energy is all-powerful. (40) Maintains order. (44) Occupies all space for all time instantaneously. (61)

Energy speed is controlled by friction, produced by atomic movements in its path. (45) The less the atom's friction, the greater the movement. Slow down energy enough and mass will be produced, transmuting energy to mass. (37, 45)

The speed of unimpeded energy is infinite. (45) Only something moving at an even greater speed would have a chance of penetration. (43)

Energy has no resistance within or without itself. (61)

In constant, immediate and complete communication with the total environment. (45)

What lies between energy and matter? (62)

Could energy be the basic pre-matter, therefore pre-atom ingredient of the universe? (41, 44)

Could there be a form of bridge through which energy and matter could move either way, representing neither true energy nor true matter? (63, 76)

Could energy, under pressure, produce a density which forms itself into transmutical atom-like structure? (45)

Could atoms be energy condensation? (45) Therefore a transitional state?

Energy-forms control atomic structure, movement, characteristics. (42)

146

Could the sun be the source of all our life energy?

Could life-energy forces come from the sun, being metabolized by the plants, producing what acupuncturists call *Ch'i*? (63) Would such Ch'i have to be metabolized?

Could the acupuncture points be the points where stale Ch'i is eliminated, creating a Ch'i cycle as with the nitrogen cycle? (64-65)

Could Ch'i, the life-force, be this pre-matter, post-energy element? (64)

Does life-force energy enter the body from the food we eat, and from the air we breathe, which is metabolized, used as a form of energy life-force, then eliminated through the acupuncture pores? (79-80)

Are there two energies, physical energy associated with food, which goes to feed the physical being, and the energy from the air which feeds the spiritual being? (82)

Could it be that acupuncture works by manipulating both energy and chemistry? (36) Should the energy be dammed up, acupuncture techniques can be used to release and regulate it. (79) Does the needle divert energy streams in the body, since metal can influence the energy flow? (94)

Is surplus Ch'i expelled through breathing, or surplus life-energy through the bowels? (80) Could metabolized surplus energy be controlled by the mechanism of the surface acupuncture points? (80)

Everything in the body functions, and it is the function that counts (69) Function being the manifestation of energy. (44)

Could this 'Energy-Matter-Bridge' relate to a static electricity type of magnetism, linking life-energy forces?

Energies involved are drawn fresh from the cosmos, and they are new and pure and healing. (81) Could the acupoints be pores of an electro-magnetic character in the skin. (97) Electro-magnetic and gravitational forces (109)

Man is an open-ended cosmic force more in tune with energy than matter. (36) Does the brain pick up vibrations, transform them into thought patterns? (46)

Could it be that, by re-zoning healthy magnetic vibrations through the organism, the energy of the body tunes into these vibrations through the organism and vibrates out the unwanted oscillations, thus permitting the chemical self-repair of the body? (110)

Index

J

Janov   72
Jennison   110
Jewel therapy   118
Judo   70, 71
Jung   72

K

Kamiya   120
Kervran, Dr. Louis C.   37, 38, 41, 50
   *Atoms can alter their structure, become
   other elements, with almost no release
   of energy*   Chapter 17 – page 123
Kilner   82
Kim Bong Han   65, Chapter 11 – page 85,
   112, 140
Kirlian   58, 59, 101
Kirlian Photography   38, 57, 58, 107
   Chapter 14 – page 101, 107
   Explanation (Inyushin)   104
   Organic matter has a changing pattern
   Inorganic matter has a constant pattern
   Synergetics   102
   Bio-energy   103
   Bio plasma   104
   Organizational, non-chaotic and
   integrated   106
Koch Postulates of Disease   92
Koig   18, 137
Koestler   40
Korth, 'The father of Acupuncture'
   in the United Kingdom   13
Kozyrev   59-60
   Time density changes   59
Kraus, Friedrich
   Vegetative system concept   33, 34
Kreiger   134
Krippner   103
Krishnamurti   50, 51, 72, 73, 74, 107
   To love is to be free   50
   To live in the here and now   50
Kushi, Michio   83
Kyungrak   85, 86-87

L

Laing   72
Lakatos   105
Lakhovsky   50, 107, 124
   (Refer 'Energy-matter-bridge')
   Chapter 9 – page 75, 77, 107, 124
Language limitations (Refer 'Energy')   9,
   43-44, 79, 94
Lao Tze   24, 25, 26, 27
   (Refer 'Tao' and 'Yin-Yang')
Laszlo   101
Lauwes   124
Lavoisier   125
Laws –
   There is nothing random in Nature   41
   Law of the Four Seasons   18
   Law of Opposites   25
   Law of entropy   125
   Law of rhythm and polarity   35
   Function controls structure   70
   Lesser sacrifice to greater   41, 69
Laws of Nature
   Disobedience   18, 20
   Negligence   19
   Rebellion   18
   Working with   90
   Understanding
Laying on of hands   37, 81, 84, 107, 110
Learning by parallel/opposite   62
Leaton   135
Lenzi   111
The lesser subordinates its needs to the greater,
   survival being the deciding factor
   41, 69, 125
Li Tan – refer Lao Tze   24
Life cycle   120
Life-energy   62, 63, 68, 70, 71, 72, 79, 80,
   84, 89, 91, 92, 106, 112, 116
   Disturbed   71
   Forces   63, 64, 67, 68, 134
   Patterns   71, 72
Life-force   17, 25, 61, 62, 67, 68, 69, 70,
   71, 72, 73, 79, 80, 81, 84, 90, 106
   Controls function   70
Life forms   72
Life forces   31, 133

Nirvana, universal   11, 71
North   82, 112, 113, 116, 136, 138
Numbness (Refer 'The five illnesses of
  numbness')   19
Nutrition   50, 70

O

Obedience to the Laws of Nature   20
Odic force   84
Open-ended system   36, 46, 103, 109
Opposites   22 (Refer 'Ch'i')
  Law of Opposites   25, 62
OR – Orgone Energy   89,
  Reich, Chapter 12 – page 89
Order   19, 25
Orgage   72
Organic food essential to health   64
Organic force   17
Organic and inorganic matter   101, 105
Organistic energy emissions   33
Organizing tendency   106
Orgone   89, 93
Orgone accumulator   89, 92, 94, 96
  Energy   33, 43, 89, 95
OR   89, 95
Orgone Therapy   53, 89
Oscillations   43, 75, 76, 110, 114, 115
  118, 135, 137, 138, 139
  *Oscillate correctly and live
  harmoniously*   75
Origin   15, 16
Osteo-arthritis   112, 113
Osteopathy   49, 72, 109
Ouspensky   72
Over-reaction initially   35
Oxygen   70, 92, 95

P

P32 (phosporus 32)   86, 87
Pain reduced   56
Palmer   137

Palpation   29
Parapsychologists   103
Parasympathetic nervous system   36
  (Refer 'vegetative')
Pavlov   33
Peace (neutral colours - blue, green, yellow)   29
  Law of Opposites   25
  Centre of spectrum   29
  Balance   29
Pendulum   36, 53, 59, 60
Peper   121
Phantom Leaf effect   102,
  (Refer Kirlian Photography)   104, 105
Phantom pulse   104
Phillipines   108
Philosophy, Tao   25, 26, 27
Photosynthesis   114
Physical structure   70
Physical-emotional-spiritual balance   50, 67
Piccardi   131
Pien Ch'iao   30-31
Piezoelectric Detector of Bioplasm   57
Pittendrigh   140
Plants,   63, 65, 71, 73, 79, 101, 106, 108,
  111, 112, 126, 127, 129, 132, 138, 141
  Plants transform inorganic energy into
  organic energy, then available for animal
  metabolism.
Point Location   56, 99
  Needling   34
Polarity   35, 59, 76, 82, 83, 112,
  113, 114, 116, 117, 138
Post-energy   44, 64, 79, 82
Prana   43, 65, 71, 79, 84
Pre-atom, post-energy   41, 44, 63, 79, 83
Pre-matter, therefore pre-atom   41, 64, 79, 82
Premises of thesis (Refer Page 146)
Presman   104-105
Pressure   22, 93
Primal Therapy   89
Pro-life   51, 52, 64, 71, 104, 112
Pro-life principles (Refer 'Health')
  Treating the whole being   50
Protein Nitrogen (increase in cell
  formation)   87
Prout   124
Provirus Theory   94